• LOW VISION •

· LOW VISION ·

A Symposium Marking the Twentieth Anniversary of The Lighthouse Low Vision Service

Edited by

ELEANOR E. FAYE, M.D., F.A.C.S.
*Medical Director
New York Lighthouse Low Vision Service
Attending Surgeon
Manhattan Eye, Ear and Throat Hospital
New York, New York*

And

CLARE M. HOOD, R.N., M.A.
*Administrative Director
New York Lighthouse Low Vision Service
New York, New York*

With a Foreword by

Wesley D. Sprague
*Executive Director
The Lighthouse
The New York Association for the Blind*

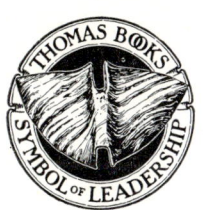

CHARLES C THOMAS · PUBLISHER
Springfield · Illinois · U.S.A.

Published and Distributed Throughout the World by
CHARLES C THOMAS • PUBLISHER
BANNERSTONE HOUSE
301-327 East Lawrence Avenue, Springfield, Illinois, U.S.A.

*This book is protected by copyright. No
part of it may be reproduced in any manner
without written permission from the publisher.*

© 1975, by CHARLES C THOMAS • PUBLISHER
ISBN 0-398-03372-2
Library of Congress Catalog Card Number: 74-26641

With **THOMAS BOOKS** *careful attention is given to all details of manufacturing and design. It is the Publisher's desire to present books that are satisfactory as to their physical qualities and artistic possibilities and appropriate for their particular use.* **THOMAS BOOKS** *will be true to those laws of quality that assure a good name and good will.*

Printed in the United States of America
H-2

Library of Congress Cataloging in Publication Data
Main entry under title:

Low vision.
    Bibliography: p.
    Includes index.
    1. Vision disorders—Congresses.   2. Ophthalmic lenses—Congresses.
3. Lighthouse Low Vision Service.
I. Faye, Eleanor E., 1923- ed. II. Hood, Clare M., ed.
III. Lighthouse Low Vision Service.
[DNLM: 1. Vision disorders—Congresses. WW100 L912 1973]
RE48.L68   617.7'12   74-26641
ISBN 0-398-03372-2

DEDICATED

to

The ophthalmologists and optometrists
and low vision technicians and assistants
who are doing clinical Low Vision.

CONTRIBUTORS

Robert J. Adrian, Ph.D.: *Psychological Coordinator, New York Association for the Blind, Associate Professor of Educational Psychology, Queens College.*

John E. Asarkof, O.D.: *Optometric Director, Vision Rehabilitation Clinic, University Hospital, Mass.*

Alan H. Barnert, M.D.: *Clinician, New York Lighthouse Low Vision Service, Attending Surgeon, Manhattan Eye, Ear and Throat Hospital.*

Norman C. Charles, M.D.: *Clinician, New York Lighthouse Low Vision Service, Clinical Assistant Professor of Ophthalmology, New York University School of Medicine.*

Eleanor E. Faye, M.D., F.A.C.S.: *Medical Director, New York Lighthouse Low Vision Service, Attending Surgeon, Manhattan Eye, Ear and Throat Hospital.*

Richard E. Feinbloom: *General Manager, Designs for Vision, Inc.*

Leslie Fine, M.D.: *Chief, Department of Psychiatry, Coney Island Hospital, New York.*

Dagmar B. Friedman, M.S.W.: *Administrative Director, Vision Rehabilitation Clinic, University Hospital, Mass.*

Arlene R. Gordon, M.S.W.: *Associate Executive Director, The New York Association for the Blind.*

Ellis Gruber, M.D.: *Director, Low Vision Clinic, Rochester Association for the Blind, Clinical Assistant Professor of Ophthalmology, University of Rochester School of Medicine, New York.*

George O. Hellinger, O.D.: *Director, Low Vision Service, Industrial Home for the Blind, New York.*

Wayne W. Hoeft, O.D.: *Director, Low Vision Service, Southern California College of Optometry.*

Clare M. Hood, R.N., M.A.: *Administrative Director, New York Lighthouse Low Vision Service, Director, Medical Services, The New York Association for the Blind.*

Randall T. Jose, O.D.: *Coordinator, Clinical Services for the Partially Sighted, School of Optometry, University of Alabama.*

Arthur H. Keeney, M.D., F.A.C.S.: *Dean, Medical School, University of Louisville.*

Dennis K. Kelleher, Ed.D, FAAO: *Clinical Instructor in Low Vision, School of Optometry, University of California, Consultant, Low Vision Services, Yolo County Schools Office.*

Joel A. Kraut, M.D., F.A.C.S.: *Director, Low Vision Center, Massachusetts Eye and Ear Infirmary, Clinical Assistant in Ophthalmology, Harvard Medical School.*

Thomas R. Kuhns, M.D., F.A.C.S.: *Clinician, New York Lighthouse Low Vision Service, Clinical Associate Professor of Ophthalmology, New York University School of Medicine.*

LoRetta McAdams, O.T.: *Optometric Technician, Low Vision Service, School of Optometry, University of Alabama.*

Kay McDonald, M.A.: *Vocational Rehabilitation Counselor, The New York Association for the Blind.*

Norman B. Medow, M.D.: *Assistant Attending Surgeon, Manhattan Eye, Ear and Throat Hospital, Assistant Attending Surgeon, Department of Ophthalmology, St. Luke's Hospital Medical Center.*

Morris J. Mintz, M.D.: *Medical Director, Low Vision Service, Sinai Hospital, Michigan.*

Charles R. Moore, M.D.: *Private Practice, Ga.*

Julian D. Newman, O.D.: *Low Vision Consultant to the Bureau of Blind Services, FL, Chairman, Clinical Examination Committee, Low Vision Diplomate Program, American Academy of Optometry.*

Contributors

Alfred A. Rosenbloom, M.A., O.D.: *President, Illinois College of Optometry.*

Boyd H. Seidenberg, M.D., F.A.C.S.: *Clinician, New York Lighthouse Low Vision Service, Clinical Instructor, Department of Ophthalmology, New York University Medical Center, Attending Ophthalmologist, Valley Hospital, N.J.*

Wesley D. Sprague, M.S.: *Executive Director, The New York Association for the Blind.*

Elisabeth Stern, R.N., B.S.: *Medical Counselor, The New York Association for the Blind.*

Gwen Kunken Sterns, M.D.: *Resident in Ophthalmology, Nassau County Medical Center, New York.*

Carter B. Tallman, M.D.: *Medical Director, Vision Rehabilitation Clinic, University Hospital, Mass.*

Sidney Weiss, M.D.: *Director, Low Vision Aid Service, Wills Eye Hospital, Pennsylvania.*

Donald B. Whitney: *Director, Product Engineering, American Optical Corporation, Massachusetts.*

Lawrence Yannuzzi, M.D.: *Associate Attending Surgeon, Manhattan Eye, Ear and Throat Hospital, Director, Fluorescein Angiography Laboratory, Manhattan Eye, Ear and Throat Hospital.*

FOREWORD

The publication of these Proceedings represents another facet of the continuing educational efforts in the field of low vision by The Lighthouse, The New York Association for the Blind.

The seminar at which these papers were presented marked the twentieth anniversary of the Lighthouse Low Vision Service, two decades devoted to examining patients, prescribing aids, and encouraging and training other professionals to expand their assistance to people with impaired vision.

The opening of the Lighthouse Low Vision Service in 1953 was a natural step for an agency which as early as 1908 had an oculist on staff who, from that time on, worked both within the agency and with physicians in the surrounding area to provide eye examinations aimed at the prevention of blindness.

Not even the visionary men and women who headed the Lighthouse at that time could have foreseen the rise of that small clinic to its present preeminent position. Dr. Conrad Berens, a leading New York ophthalmologist who served on the Lighthouse Board of Directors, was fortunate in persuading Dr. Gerald Fonda to survey the first five hundred patients. It was Dr. Fonda who brought in Dr. Alfred Kestenbaum, the pioneer Viennese ophthalmologist. He, in turn, developed the Mikroscopic lens which introduced the concept of special lenses for low vision that were not telescopic and which revolutionized the field.

It was due to the efforts of these men and Dr. Eleanor E. Faye, who became medical director in 1966, that the influence of the Lighthouse Low Vision Service went far beyond clinical service to clients. With the example of hundreds and then thousands of men and women who were restored to varying degrees of functional vision by prescription and training in the use of special lenses by a skilled supporting staff, they were able to interest more and more of their colleagues in the field. When technical advances in plastics made possible the manufacture of high strength lenses with a better field than those made in glass, the Low Vision Service was instrumental in getting optical companies involved in developing better and more appropriate devices.

Over the years the Lighthouse Low Vision Service has trained 650 physicians and their assistants in low vision work, 225 of these being residents in ophthalmology from eleven New York City hospitals. In addition it has helped establish low vision clinics throughout the U.S. and abroad, and it has played an active role in founding the Low Vision Clinical Society whose annual section meeting is prior to that of the American Academy of Ophthalmology and Otolaryngology.

Staff members regularly participate in medical meetings throughout the country and have developed special exhibit material for these sessions. Two teaching films, a video tape, and a textbook on the low vision patient represent the clinical experience of the Low Vision Service.

In the research area, the Lighthouse Low Vision Service has itself developed several lenses, test kits, and vision testing charts in addition to its work with optical companies. It has the largest central distribution center of optical aids in the country for low vision specialists and clinics.

Despite the justifiable pride The Lighthouse takes in these accomplishments, there is still much to be done in all these areas. The papers presented at the seminar direct attention to the research and standards of practice needed to insure that all with failing vision can get the most use from what sight they have left. Private and public agencies, together with practitioners in the community, must share this responsibility.

Wesley D. Sprague, M.S.
Executive Director
The New York Association for the Blind

PREFACE

Visual impairment is a subject which has for decades intrigued ophthalmologists and optometrists with a special bent toward optics. The pioneers such as Kestenbaum, Feinbloom, Fonda, and Linksz were interested in and developed devices which were ingenious. Their writings were largely overlooked by all but the most dedicated refractionists who realized that a certain group of patients was not getting good clinical care except in a very specialized and limited sense.

In the past few years there has been an upsurge of interest throughout the eye professions in what amounts to a clinical revival. Numerous clinics have been started, and the trend has been to move away from the solo practitioner toward the clinic with all of its services needed by the person who has suffered a visual loss with its allied economic, social, and psychological problems. No longer is Low Vision a pair of spectacles, a hand magnifier, or a telescope. We now recognize the complex person who must wear these devices in order to approximate what he once knew as normal sight or to make up for what he never had in his life. We now appreciate the fact that vision, no matter how impaired, gives ample clues for function, and lenses can help people use their residual vision, not restore them to *normal,* but amplify the clues and bring visual material to their eyes and brains.

In assembling the speakers for the Lighthouse Low Vision Service's Twentieth Anniversary, an attempt was made to highlight new subjects (advances in lens technology, new uses for lenses and nonoptical devices, advances in medical and surgical treatment of eye disease) and to discuss frankly such a controversial subject as driving with telescopes. We tried to include practical clinical material on the visual problems of all the age groups; the child, the young adult who is still in the vocational years, and the elderly person. We have included some interesting neurological material and touched on the complex subject of prisms and mirrors. The accent is on clinical experience rather than an extensive review of the literature. The few references at the end of each author's chapter are included as a source of further reading of worthwhile material.

Finally, we have included a section devoted to the organizational patterns of several clinics in the hope that they can serve as models for other clinics. We have also included a valuable section suggesting a training curriculum for the Low Vision assistant and suggesting future direction in the field.

The most unusual feature of the Symposium was the variety of professional credits of a group representing ophthalmologists, optometrists, rehabilitation counselors, social workers, nurses, and optical designers. This *is* the trend in the field of Low Vision: cooperation on a clinical and academic level among all these people for the sake of the patients with subnormal vision. We hope that this book will provide material applicable to the interests and skills of every professional person interested in Low Vision.

Eleanor E. Faye, M.D.

ACKNOWLEDGMENTS

The Lighthouse Low Vision Service is greatly indebted to the New York Association for the Blind (The Lighthouse) for supporting us in an atmosphere in which constant growth, reevaluation, and progress could be maintained. The entire staff from the executives to the clerks has been helpful and encouraging in our attempts to provide the best patient care possible.

We are also indebted to the Barth Foundation for a generous annual donation which has allowed us to develop educational programs and exhibits at the American Academy of Ophthalmology and Otolaryngology since December, 1968. Their support has enabled us to investigate new lenses, improve our patient care, and to organize the 20th Anniversary Symposium on an appropriate scale.

Special thanks are due the Low Vision Assistants, the clinic nurses who helped organize the details of the Symposium, and to our Lighthouse volunteers in the medical service who helped do the many tasks that made the Symposium run smoothly.

We are grateful to the American Optical Company for their assistance.

We thank the typists from the volunteer and word processing departments of the Lighthouse who coped with new technical words in the overwhelming number of manuscripts that had to be prepared.

We thank our photographer Andrew Gordon for his technical assistance at the Symposium and his excellent photographs of aids and Tony Lobacz for his excellent photographs and prints of optical aids.

We also could not have managed all of the many details which Margaret Marcone handled with such tact and skill.

E.E.F.
C.M.H.

CONTENTS

	Page
Contributors	vii
Foreword	xi
Preface	xiii
Acknowledgments	xv

SECTION ONE—OPTICAL AND NONOPTICAL AIDS

Chapter

    I. PRACTICAL USES FOR SPECTACLES AND SIMPLE MAGNIFIERS—Eleanor E. Faye 5

    II. TELESCOPIC SYSTEMS—Julian D. Newman 17

    III. TREATING SUBNORMAL VISION IN APHAKIA—Charles R. Moore 31

    IV. CLOSED CIRCUIT TELEVISION: ITS VALUE IN LOW VISION—Morris J. Mintz 37

    V. NONOPTICAL AIDS—Clare M. Hood 42

SECTION TWO—DEVELOPMENT OF VISUAL AIDS

    VI. THE OPTICAL DESIGN OF SPECTACLE MAGNIFIERS—Donald B. Whitney 51

    VII. FUTURE DEVELOPMENT OF OPTICAL AIDS—Richard E. Feinbloom 60

SECTION THREE—SURGICAL AND MEDICAL ADVANCES IN OPHTHALMOLOGY RELATED TO THE LOW VISION PATIENT

    VIII. LATEST ADVANCES IN OPHTHALMIC SURGERY: IMPLICATIONS FOR THE LOW VISION PATIENT—Norman B. Medow 71

Chapter	Page
IX. Laser Treatment and Low Vision Anatomical Considerations—Norman C. Charles	79
X. Argon Laser Coagulation (ALC)—Lawrence Yannuzzi	87

SECTION FOUR—FIELD DEFECTS AND OPTICAL MANAGEMENT

XI. Neuro-Ophthalmological Defects in the Partially Sighted Patient— Thomas R. Kuhns	97
XII. Mirrors, Prisms, and Eccentric Field Defects—Wayne W. Hoeft	103

SECTION FIVE—VISION REHABILITATION FROM CHILDHOOD TO THE VOCATIONAL YEARS

XIII. Pediatric Low Vision—Boyd H. Seidenberg	117
XIV. Psychological Evaluation of Low Vision Patients Using Closed Circuit Television—Robert J. Adrian	130
XV. Low Vision Patients in Vocational Rehabilitation Programs—Elisabeth Stern	137
XVI. Rehabilitation Using Aids: Modification During Vocational Training—Kay McDonald	141
XVII. Cases in Which Optical Aids Made a Crucial Difference—George O. Hellinger	146

SECTION SIX—VISION REHABILITATION IN THE GERIATRIC POPULATON

XVIII. The Older Visually Limited Person: A Statistical Profile—Arlene R. Gordon	159
XIX. Community Programs for the Visually Impaired Geriatric Patient—Leslie Fine	164

Chapter		Page
XX.	CARE OF THE ELDERLY LOW VISION PATIENT: EVALUATION, AIDS, PROGNOSTIC FACTORS—Alfred A. Rosenbloom	169

SECTION SEVEN—DRIVING WITH TELESCOPES

XXI.	THE RATIONALE FOR LICENSURE: CRITERIA AND TRAINING—Julian D. Newman	179
XXII.	A POSITIVE APPROACH TO DRIVING WITH TELESCOPIC GLASSES—Carter B. Tallman	183
XXIII.	EXPERIENCE OF A LOW VISION PATIENT DRIVING WITH A BIOPTIC TELESCOPE—Dennis K. Kelleher	189
XXIV.	A CAUTIONARY VIEW OF DRIVING WITH TELESCOPES—George O. Hellinger	199
XXV.	OPERATIONAL LIMITATIONS OF DRIVING WITH TELESCOPES—Arthur H. Keeney and Sidney Weiss	204
XXVI.	DISCUSSION OF DRIVING CRITERIA—Alan H. Barnert	208

SECTION EIGHT—MODELS OF LOW VISION CLINICS

XXVII.	LOW VISION CLINICS: THE NEED, THE ORGANIZATION, THE MANPOWER—Randall T. Jose	215
XXVIII.	A LOW VISION PROGRAM IN ROCHESTER, NEW YORK—Ellis Gruber	220
XXIX.	THE VISION REHABILITATION CLINIC AT BOSTON UNIVERSITY MEDICAL CENTER—	
	THE ROLE OF THE OPHTHALMOLOGIST—Carter B. Tallman	228
	THE ROLE OF THE SOCIAL WORKER—Dagmar B. Friedman	234
XXX.	THE LOW VISION CLINIC: UNIVERSITY OF ALABAMA SCHOOL OF OPTOMETRY—Randall T. Jose and LoRetta McAdams	241

Chapter	Page
XXXI. The Lighthouse Low Vision Service (New York)—Eleanor E. Faye and Clare M. Hood	253

SECTION NINE—TRAINING PROGRAMS IN LOW VISION CLINICS

XXXII. Instruction of the Ophthalmology Resident: Massachusetts Eye and Ear Infirmary—Joel Kraut	267
XXXIII. A Resident's View of Low Vision Training—Gwen K. Sterns	273
XXXIV. A Training Program for the Low Vision Technician—Randall T. Jose	276
Index	285

• LOW VISION •

· SECTION ONE ·

Optical and Nonoptical Aids

· CHAPTER I ·
Practical Uses for Spectacles and Simple Magnifiers

Eleanor E. Faye

LET US consider for a moment what happens to a person when his normal vision is impaired. The normal eye has the spontaneous ability to see everything at once and make a rapid visual choice. To the diseased eye the surroundings look distorted, blurred, or incomplete. Viewing objects becomes a deliberate task which requires either some type of optical aid or some form of amplification of the image. Visual spontaneity is lost. The laborious process of learning to use this impaired vision starts with a tangible optical aid, a pair of glasses or a magnifier, which can help the person believe with his own eyes that he has usable vision. No efforts at rehabilitation or restoration of confidence will work until the patient grasps the new image of himself as a person who will *never* see well again, who must learn to use what he has effectively, and who must use an optical aid nearly every time he wants to see things in detail.

While Low Vision may mean *glasses* to a patient, to the doctor who does low vision work it means keeping up with the multiplicity of aids that are now available and knowing how to prescribe them. A knowledge of simple optical principles will help him decide whether to prescribe a spectacle, a telescopic loupe, a hand magnifier, or a combination of these aids for reading and close work. He must also be aware of patients' activities *other* than reading and use his imagination to think of variations in aids for unusual needs.

Since the principal goal is to provide optical compensation for a wide range of visual activities, multiple types of aids are a necessity to fill each gap in visual function for the patient. To fall into the exclusive use of one type of aid is potentially to neglect the patient's needs and limit his adjustment.

Simple aids, that is, spectacles alone, hand magnifiers alone, and combinations of the two solve over 85 percent of the prescription needs for the patient. This chapter will discuss some unusual clinical uses for these aids. For patients whose needs exceed the limitations of simple aids, the examiner must have more sophisticated knowledge of microscopic systems and telescopic lenses discussed in the following chapters.

Optical devices fall into three general categories: spectacle (headborne) lenses, hand held lenses, or telescopic lenses. For people new to low vision work, the use of simple lenses in spectacles and hand held devices should precede the use of the telescope, a more complex aid.

The Low Vision Examination

One of the objectives of the low vision examination is to present the patient with a positive approach to his residual vision. The first step in giving a patient confidence in his vision is an accurate, carefully taken visual acuity. The vision chart is best held within the functional range of the patient, ten to five feet away. The acuity measurement is used in its inverse ratio as a useful indicator of the numbers of diopters needed in the low vision aid for the patient to read average print. Known as the Kestenbaum Formula, this simple calculation can be done on any visual acuity, taken at any distance, with any numerical system. It is not a foolproof calculation because the patient's visual function is often at odds with his *acuity*. The magnification factor may have to be adjusted during the examination as the patient's abilities and needs are clarified.

After the amount of needed correction has been established, test the patient's reaction to a high plus add.[1] Some examiners find it easier to work with props, that is, with aids already made up in frames. For the patient to wear the actual aid when he is reading is far more realistic because he sees what his final aid will be like. He can decide if he feels comfortable with the aid rather than leaving the choice up to the examiner.

If the patient rejects the close working distance of the spectacle, the examiner can safely retreat to a hand magnifier, realizing something about the patient; that he may not be able to cope with high magnification yet. Many experienced examiners at this point would prescribe a telescopic loupe to gain working distance, but it is worth considering the clinical evidence that a patient who cannot accept spectacle magnification also cannot cope with the restrictive features of a telescope. It might be more roundabout to use a hand magnifier as a training device, but the patient's acceptance is more secure. Flexibility of prescription is of increasing interest to the low vision practitioner. Practical methods of using different approaches will be amplified in the following paragraphs.

Half-eye Lenses

An acceptable alternative to a full spectacle is the half-eye glass, with 6, 8, or 10 diopters with compensating base-in prism in each eye to help both eyes converge.[2] The half-eye glasses with prism provide binocular reading vision for patients with relatively moderate vision loss and potential binocularity. The stock glasses are manu-

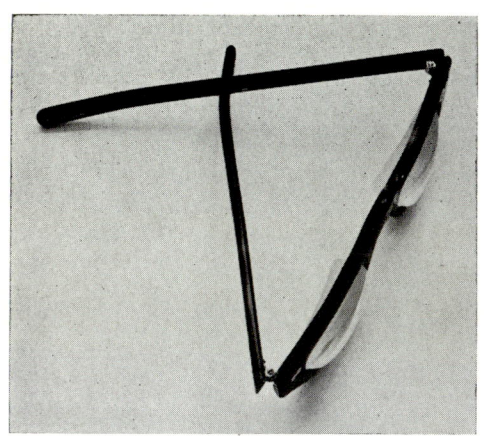

Figure I-1. A half-eye frame for high power lenses allows unobstructed distance vision. Glasses are premounted in a choice of 6-, 8- or 10-diopter lenses with prism base-in to aid convergence.

factured only up to 10 diopters, which means that they are worth a trial for patients within the better acuity range from 20/40 to 20/200. These patients tend to have diseases with limited pathology such as early macular degeneration, early diabetes, moderate cataracts, or a variety of congenital diseases of the macula, retina, and optic nerve. They adapt well to this comfortable aid and do not object to its cosmetic appearance. For well-motivated patients who need a + 12 add and can use lenses *binocularly*, American Optical Company can make up a special lens using Fresnel prisms to provide the full 16 diopters of prism base-in needed for convergence. The half-eye prism glasses can use a monocular lens of any strength, and even a lenticular can be cut to conform to the frame shape. The use of the half-eye glass is flexible. It may be used three ways: alone, over the present correction, or in combination with a hand magnifier.

If it is used alone and if the patient has no other refractive error, it may be preferable to a bifocal. If the patient is myopic, his uncorrected eye will give additional power to the lens; for example, if the refractive error were -4.00 diopters, the 8-diopter reading glass over the uncorrected eye would give an effective add of 12 diopters.

Conversely, if the patient is basically hyperopic, the reading add is reduced unless the patient slips the half-glass on over the distance prescription. The half-glass can also be slipped on over a bifocal,

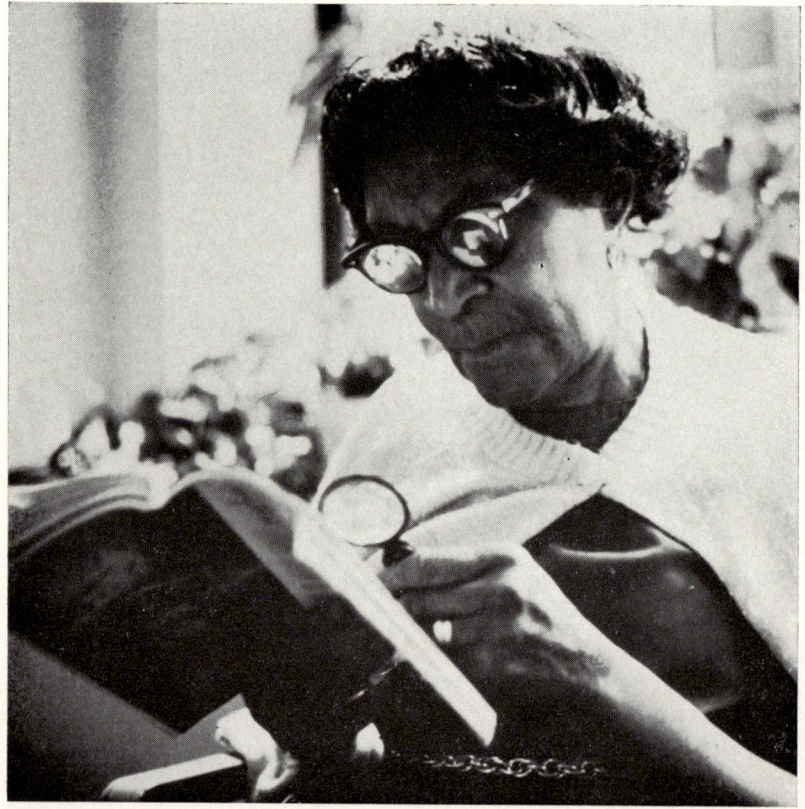

Figure I-2. When a patient objects to reading too close with a spectacle, the add may be divided between the spectacle and a hand magnifier.

if the patient is accustomed to wearing a bifocal. He then has the advantage of a little extra correction; for example, an add of 3 diopters combines with the 10-diopter glass to give a total add of 13 diopters. Used in this way the range of the 6, 8, or 10 diopters is increased.

The third method of using the half-glass with a hand magnifier will serve to illustrate two important concepts: splitting the add and prescribing a lower add geared to seeing larger print. Splitting a high add between the spectacle and hand magnifier means using 4, 5, 6, or 8 diopters in the spectacle. This extends the reading distance to that of the weaker spectacle lens. For example, a patient might not be able to tolerate a 14-diopter add with its reading distance of less than three inches. By putting 6 of the diopters in the half-glass, the reading distance is extended to 6½ inches, and an 8 D hand magnifier provides the same total add. The patient is getting the same magnification with more ease and comfort. Another flexible arrangement can be made by using the patient's own standard bifocal or prescribing a slightly higher add (up to 5 D is available without a special order) to be used with higher powers of hand magnifiers.

The second concept is to prescribe one of the half-glasses which will be adequate for regular or large print only. When small type or detailed vision is required, a supplementary hand magnifier can be added. By using the half-glass this way as a base, many different strengths of hand magnifiers can be introduced particularly for patients with varied interests and needs. Keeler [2] manufactures a type of half lens, a full vision lens with a small crescent segment cut out of the top rim that allows the same type of unobstructed distance vision as the half-eye frame. They are for monocular use only and come in strengths of 2x, 3x, 4x, 6x, and 8x.

Full-vision Lenses

When patients have poor enough eyesight to require 12 to 20 diopters of add (20/120 to 20/300 approximately), they more easily accept a full-vision lens. They need the larger field, and distance vision is not as important. The examiner will obtain more precise reactions with the full lenses premounted in frames (identical lenses for OD and OS so that either eye can be tested monocularly.) The eye not in use can be occluded with a plastic or Keeler clip-on occluder to eliminate distracting impressions. Use plastic aspheric standard lenses from 12 diopters to 20 diopters. Above 20 D use special microscopic lenses which are manufactured by several companies. There are 24 D and 32 D Igard and A.O. plastic lenses. Special high add bifocals may be prescribed for the patient who prefers them, who has a significant refractive error (an aphakic patient for example), or who needs them for a job.

Designs for Vision, Keeler, and the American Optical Company manufacture a complete line of special lenses, and trial sets are available.

Magnifiers

The optical advantages of a spectacle aid may be a disadvantage to the patient. He may have both hands free and the widest possible field of any aid, but he has to adjust to a very close, fixed reading distance of eight inches or less. Here, the hand magnifier will have a distinct advantage.

Hand magnifiers are the most common, the most acceptable, and the most flexible aid. They should be rescued from haphazard

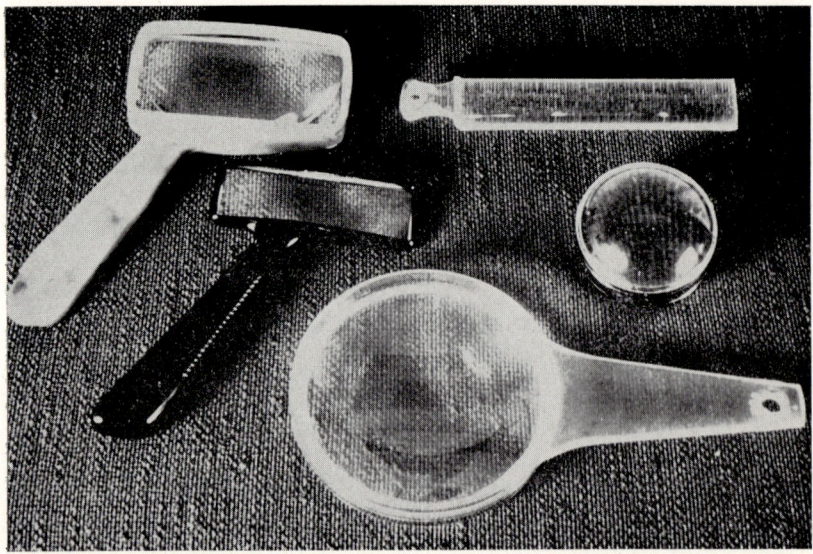

Figure I-3. Hand and stand magnifiers in the 5-diopter range.

Practical Uses for Spectacles and Simple Magnifiers 11

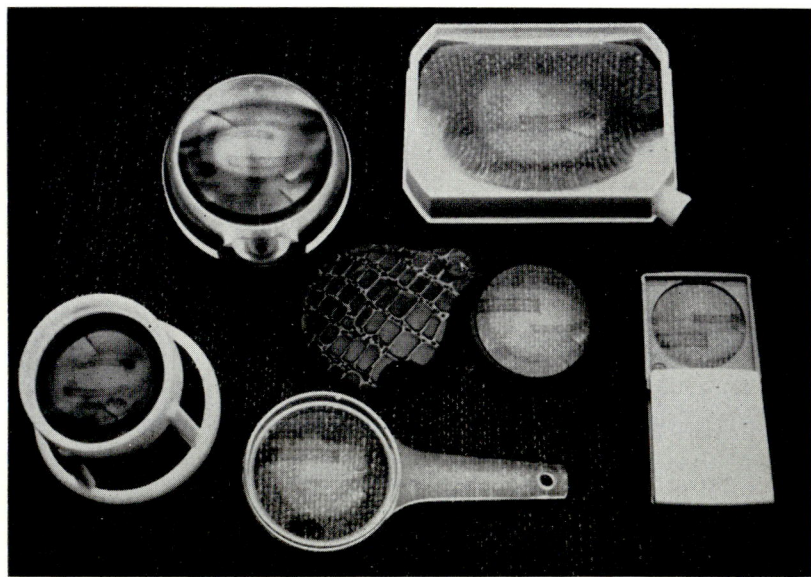

Figure I-4. Hand and stand magnifiers in the 7 to 12-diopter range.

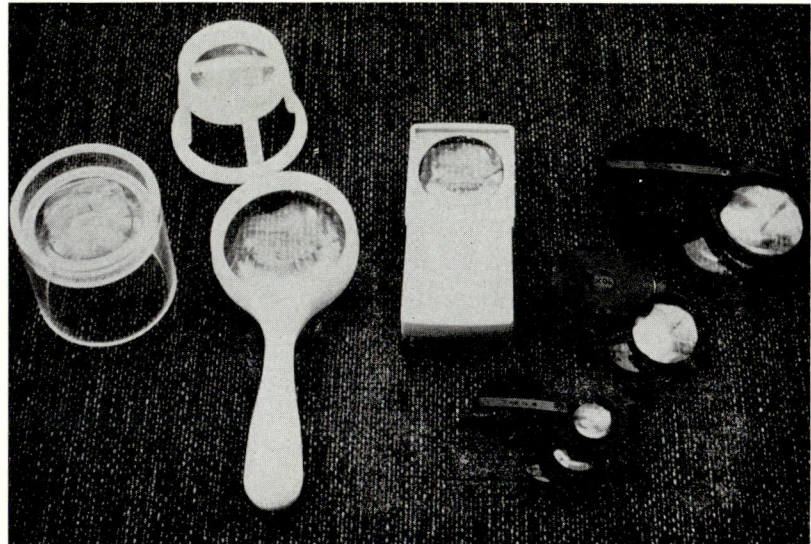

Figure I-5. Hand and stand magnifiers in the 20 to 67-diopter range.

prescription and from the slightly condescending attitude often expressed toward this humble and versatile aid. In the gamut of hand magnifiers, selection should be somewhat restricted to avoid confusion. The most commonly used and accepted magnifiers in the 5 D range include the Edroy, B&L, COIL and Selsi.[2] These lenses are used by people with minimal vision loss. The 7 D and 12 D COIL, the Selsi +11, and the B&L +11[2] are used by patients who have a moderate loss in the area of 20/200 or perhaps 20/300. For those with more severe vision loss, the 20 D COIL, the B&L 5x, 7x, and 20x, and the 10x Selsi are acceptable.[2]

The greatest advantage of the hand magnifier seems to be its acceptance as a familiar aid in everyday use by all kinds of people. The transition that a person who is losing sight has to make is easier with an aid that is not so strange or frightening.

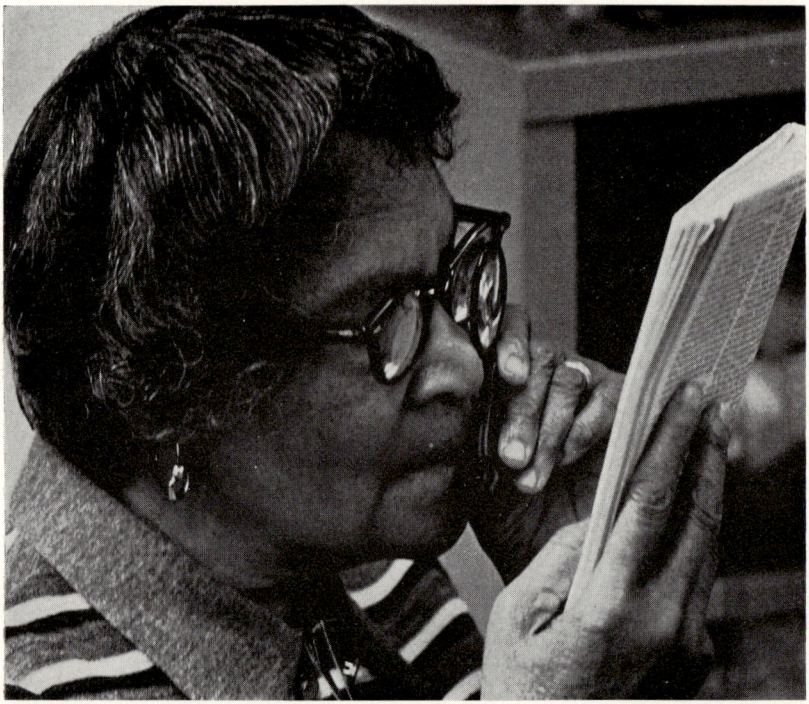

Figure I-6. A hand magnifier may be held against the glasses to increase the magnification quickly for small print. It is used to train patients to accept high magnification.

Practical Uses for Spectacles and Simple Magnifiers

The greatest optical advantage is that, although the lens must be held at a fixed distance from the reading material, the combination can be held at a greater distance from the eye.

There are other advantages to this versatile aid. The magnifier can be moved closer to the eye or held against the glasses. This combination as a training method often teaches the patient the *spectacle effect* without his being aware of it. He may spontaneously ask if the combination could be made up in a reading glass after he has used it for awhile, and because it is his own idea, he adjusts to it.

Patients think up many uses for hand magnifiers. They check the labels on cans, bottles of pills, prices on foods and clothing. They need to read directions, recipes, thermostats, thermometers, oven and refrigerator settings. They can keep up their independence by reading menus, circulars, phone numbers. Some patients have discovered that they can also use a hand magnifier as a stand. It can be done with any magnifier with a wide rim (COIL 8 D).

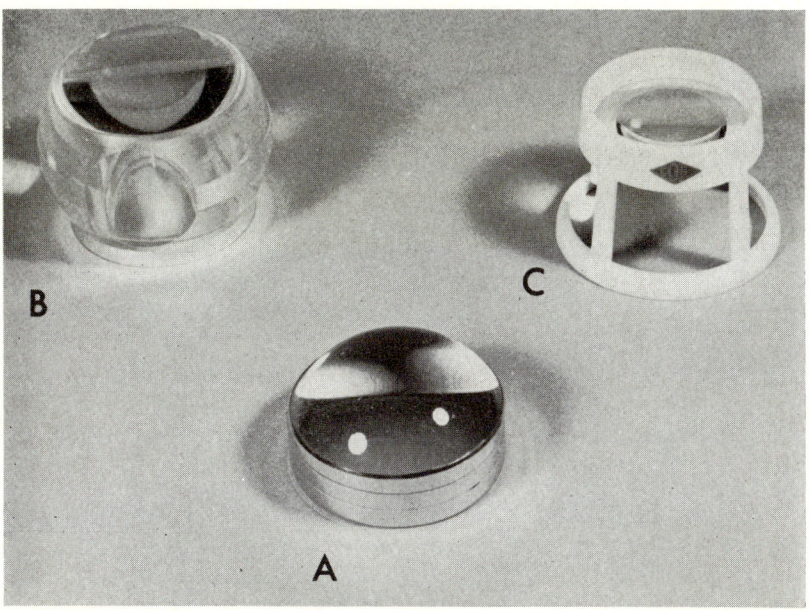

Figure I-7. Three useful prefocused stand magnifiers are (a) planoconvex 4.7D, (b) Jupiter 9D, (c) COIL 17.6D.

Stand Magnifier

The stand magnifier is a neglected aid, often forgotten by the doctor and discovered by the patient in his consultations with other similarly afflicted patients. On the examining table within reach should be a small selection of the stand magnifiers most often used by patients, the planoconvex Selsi, the Jupiter, and the 17 D COIL.[2] In some cases they are the aid of choice, often in the late stages of glaucoma or in eccentric field losses. It has become a convention to think of stand magnifiers as being used by people with hand tremors and arthritis. Clinically it appears that people with tremors do better with spectacles, but with arthritis the stands are easier to hold. Many older people who read the newspaper on the flat surface of a table use one

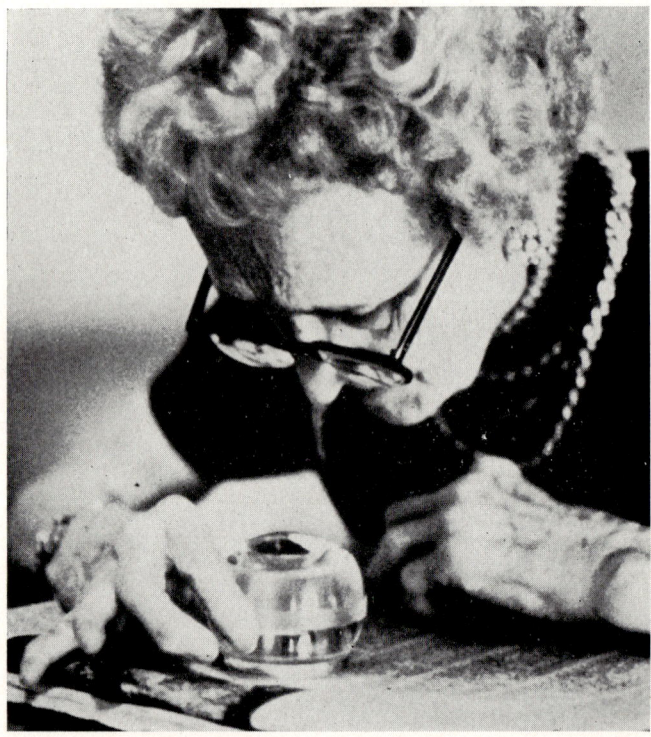

Figure I-8. A person with severe arthritis can slide a stand magnifier across a page with less fatigue than he can hold a book or paper close to the eyes.

Practical Uses for Spectacles and Simple Magnifiers

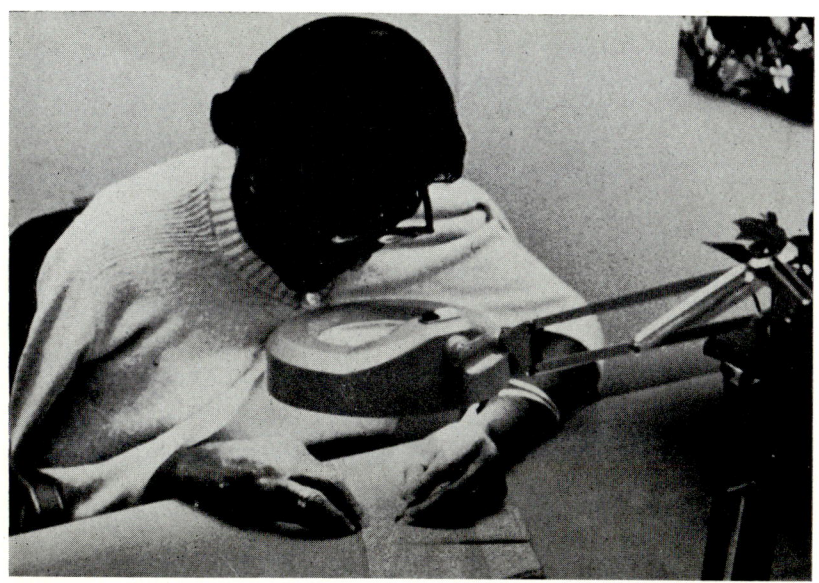

Figure I-9. The Luxo lamp has a lens insert which is particularly good for writing and keeping accounts.

of these stands. The light-gathering quality of the planoconvex lens and Jupiter stand is excellent.

The significant optical property of the fixed stand is that a patient must have 2.5 diopters of accommodation to converge the divergent rays coming from the stand. If he has insufficient accommodation, he must have a 2.5-diopter reading add. Also, except for the planoconvex stand, the amount of add than can be used with the nonadjustable stand is usually no more than 4 diopters. Other types of fixed stands with a self-contained light source are the 12 D or 16 D made by COIL and the 22 D Adisco.[2]

There are two other simple aids which can be overlooked in our zeal to provide complex prescriptions for our patients. Patients accept the Luxo or Dazor lens with its own fluorescent light source as a good aid for reading and writing. For anyone who sews, or knits, or does needlepoint the 5 D chest magnifier is a welcome addition.

Summary

In summary, it takes many types of aids to compensate for the

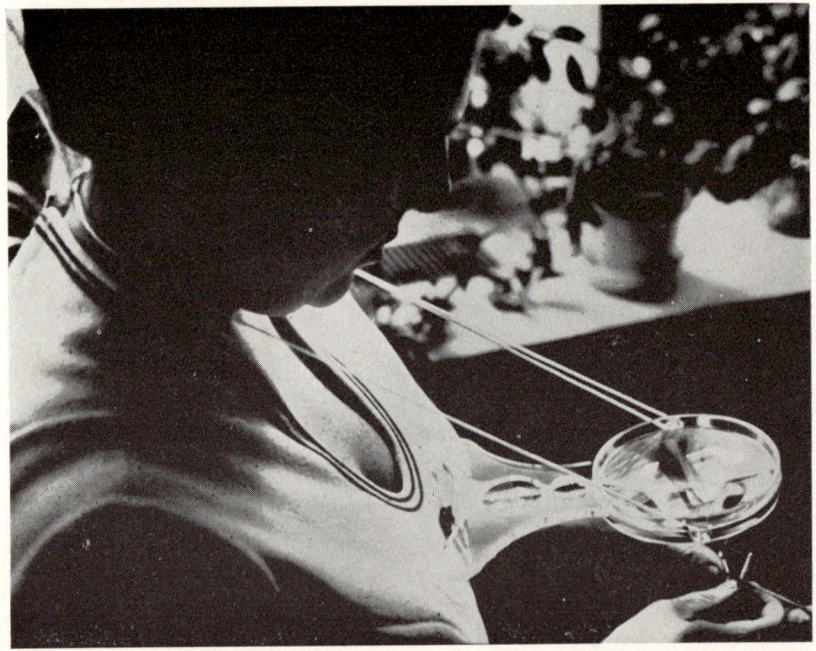

Figure I-10. This is a simple, useful aid for people who want to sew and knit. Many patients are interested in other activities than reading.

single sensory loss of vision. The characteristics and some of the unusual uses of simple aids available to the low vision patient have been discussed.

REFERENCES

1. Faye, Eleanor E.: *The Low Vision Patient.* New York, Grune and Stratton, 1970.
2. *Catalogue of Optical Aids*, 3rd ed. rev., New York, New York Lighthouse Low Vision Service, 1973.

· CHAPTER II ·
Telescopic Systems

Julian D. Newman

Introduction

THE SIMPLEST and most practical approach to the improvement of distance vision for the low vision patient is to move the object closer to the patient or the patient closer to the object. When this approach is used there is no optical distortion, no limitation of the field of view, no chromatic aberration, and no loss of contrast of the image. However, when the distance between the viewer and the object of regard is basically fixed and the viewer is a low vision patient, an optical system such as a telescope must be used to enlarge the image.

For the low vision practitioner, the telescope is also extremely useful as a diagnostic aid. The low vision practitioner will most probably use a telescopic trial lens during the refraction and may later prescribe some form of telescopic low vision aid. Therefore, the clinician should have some basic knowledge of the optics of telescopes.

The Optics of Telescopes

The telescopic system which is used in the telescopic trial lenses and most often in low vision telescopic prescriptions is the Galilean type of telescope. This type of telescope gives an erect magnified image. It consists of a convex objective lens and a concave ocular lens which is most often separated by an air space. The convex objective lens is of lower power than the concave ocular lens.

The objective and ocular lenses are placed along the optical axis and separated so that the focal plane of the anterior plus lens coincides with the virtual focal plane of the minus lens. Thus, parallel rays of light entering the system leave in a parallel manner because the system is afocal and has no refracting power. However, the system does change the angle (angle of emergence) of the parallel ray bundle by increasing this angle. Therefore, the relationship between the increase in the angle of emergence and the angle of incidence as measured along the optical axis is what creates the increase in apparent image size.

Designing a Galilean telescope to be used for the low vision patient creates certain problems for the optical designer. First of all it must be small in size and cosmetically acceptable. The system must have

1. Adequate magnification.
2. Wide field of view.
3. Only limited amounts of optical aberrations such as
    a. Chromatic aberration.
    b. Oblique astigmatism.
    c. Curvature of field.
    d. Coma.

Another optical consideration for a low vision telescope is that the exit pupil of the telescopic system must be large enough to use the full aperture of the patient's own pupil, thus insuring maximum field of view for any given system. The size of the field of view is dependent upon the degree of magnification, the size of the entrance pupil, the size of the exit pupil, separation of lenses, distance held from eye, and size of patient's pupil.

Still another problem that occurs in using an optical system such as a telescope is a diminution of light transmission as light passes through the telescopic system. This diminution occurs because of the thickness of the lenses and the number of lens surfaces. Each lens surface diminishes the light passing through the system by 4 percent.

Telescopes can also be used for intermediate and near distances by simply adding a plus lens of sufficient power to focus at the near working distance in front of the objective lens of the system. As the power of the plus lens added to the front of the objective lens increases in power, so does the total magnification of the system. However, although the magnification increases, this is accompanied by a reduction in the size of the visual field and a reduction in the working distance as well as a decrease in the depth of focus.

Using A Telescopic Trial Lens in the Low Vision Examination

At the completion of the subjective refraction of the low vision patient, a 2.2x T.S. (Telescope) trial lens should be added to the trial frame for two purposes:

1. To rerefract behind the telescope in the trial frame in order to check the accuracy of the spherical refraction.
2. To see if the patient responds positively to magnification.

A central macular lesion reduces the visual acuity; however, if the image is magnified and projected on an intact paramacular area, the image can be seen.

Thus, if the telescopic trial lens is put in place in the front cell of the trial frame, more optotypes on the visual acuity card will be discernable and more choices can be made that give the examiner the opportunity to double check the accuracy of the spherical refraction. This is done by adding plus or minus spheres to the rear cell of the trial frame. A refractive change greater than an increase in plus by $+1.00$ D or an increase in minus by $-.50$ D should be found before changing the distance subjective prescription. A cross-cylinder test with the telescopic trial lens in place is very difficult; however, the trial frame can be placed close to the face, with the telescope in the front cell. The cross cylinder is placed behind the telescope for power only. Axis is best using an astigmatic dial at 5 feet to 10 feet. If a cross-cylinder is used in front of the telescope, the telescopic system increases the effective power of the cross cylinder to the point that the test becomes too gross.

The second purpose of the telescope is to see if the patient responds to magnification. If a patient cannot read smaller optotypes when a telescopic trial lens is introduced and the patient has been properly instructed to move his head slowly and fixate on the acuity chart, most often he has a very dense central lesion or a severely constricted field. In a case such as this, measurement of the size and location of the central lesion should be made. In most cases, if there is no improvement in distance vision with magnification, there will be no improvement in near vision.

Telescopic Prescriptions

The most basic objection to the use of telescopic lenses is that the field of view decreases as the power of the magnification increases; therefore, in certain high power telescopic lenses the field of view might be only 2 or 3 degrees.

This discussion of telescopic lens systems for the low vision patient will include
  1. Head-borne fixed and variable focus telescopes.
  2. Hand-held variable focus telescopes.
  3. Contact lens telescopes.
  4. Binoculars.
  5. Telemicroscopes.
  6. Unusual types of telescopes.

The telescopes that will be discussed are generally small in size and generally low powered.

HEADBORNE FIXED AND VARIABLE FOCUS TELESCOPES: The only telescopic lens that allows the normal use of the peripheral field when viewing through the telescope is the Bioptic type of telescope (Designs for Vision and Keeler). In other types of full diameter telescopic lenses the patient has no peripheral vision.

The Designs for Vision 1.7x Bioptic has a field of approximately 26° horizontally and 21° vertically and is nonfocusable. The 2.2x Bioptic model I has a field of 12° horizontally and 9° vertically and is nonfocusable. In both cases the telescope is a small scope set in the upper portion of the lens in a normal spectacle frame. The patient's distance prescription is in the carrier portion of the lens and is also included in the telescopic portion. There is no interference with the patient's peripheral field. The whole system is light in weight and is acceptable cosmetically. The 2.2x Designs Bioptic II is smaller in size with a smaller field of 10° but is more cosmetically acceptable. The 2.2x Designs' TS Wide Angle has a much larger field, 17° horizontally and 9° vertically, but may be objectionable cosmetically. All of the aforementioned Bioptics can be used in classroom situations or for driving. The 2.2x Bioptic I can be used for driving, but the wide angle lens is preferable.

The 3x Designs' Bioptic has a clear field of 8°. It is cosmetically

Telescopic Systems

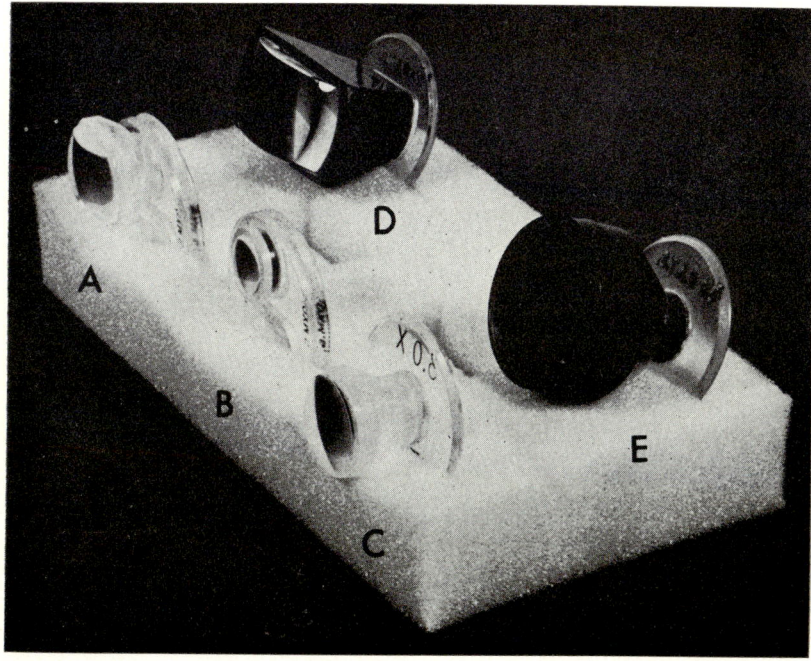

Figure II-1. Five telescopic lenses which are designed to be used in a spectacle frame (Designs for Vision): (a) 2.2x Bioptic I; (b) 2.2x Bioptic II; (c) 3x Bioptic; (d) 2.2x wide angle telescope; (e) 3x wide angle telescope.

acceptable. The 3x Designs' Wide Angle telescope has a field of 11°. It is a larger unit. Both can be used in the classroom and for driving.

The 4x Bioptic and 6x Bioptic have much smaller fields; the 4x field is 6° and the 6x Bioptic is 2°. They offer little advantage over the 6x-8x Selsi monocular other than freeing the hand which holds the monocular.

Bioptic lenses present a special problem. Most low vision patients do not have binocular vision; nevertheless, the alignment of the Bioptic type of telescopic system is critical and must be done by a very sensitive method in order to attain the situation at which the optical axis of the system and the visual axis of the patient coincide. A Bioptic is fitted on both eyes only when the visual acuity in both eyes is approximately equal, otherwise it is fit monocularly on the better eye.

Another system available is the 2.5x and 2.8x focusable binocular sportocular worn over the patient's prescription. The unit is very heavy and cosmetically objectionable. Monocularly the field of this unit is 9.5°.

Systems with the lower magnifications of 3x are generally best suited for patients with acuities of the 20/120 level, although those with magnifications of 6x are functional for those with acuities as low as 20/240.

Telescopes with magnifications of less than 3x would best be used by patients with acuities of 20/120 or better and would be best suited to situations such as the classroom in which the distance between the object and the viewer is not excessive. However, one must be aware that the distance at which he views may be commensurately increased if the best corrected visual acuity of the viewer is significantly better than 20/120.

HAND-HELD VARIABLE FOCUS TELESCOPES: The Selsi 2.5x has a field of 10° and is focusable. It is much more conspicuous. It can also be slipped over a pair of spectacles but is very heavy and may be better used hand held. Selsi also comes in a 2.8x hand held unit.

The Emoskop is a 2.5x monocular, 1¾ inches long, and focusable by sliding action. It has a 10° field and is very cosmetically acceptable.

Another telescope in this category is the ring telescope, approximately 2x. This telescope is worn on the finger as a ring and is cosmetically

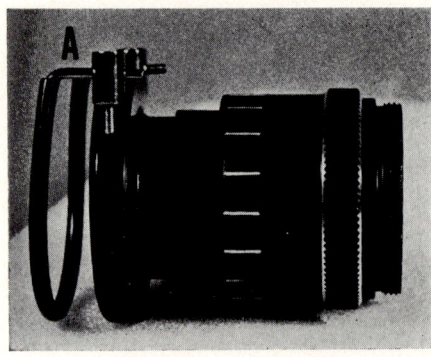
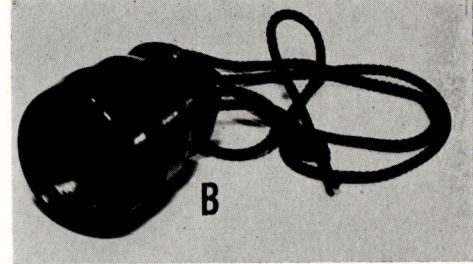

Figure II-2. (A) Clip-on Selsi 2.5x telescope may also be hand held. It is an excellent inexpensive aid for children. (B) The 2.8x Selsi monocular is lightweight, has excellent optics and sufficient magnification to be useful.

Telescopic Systems

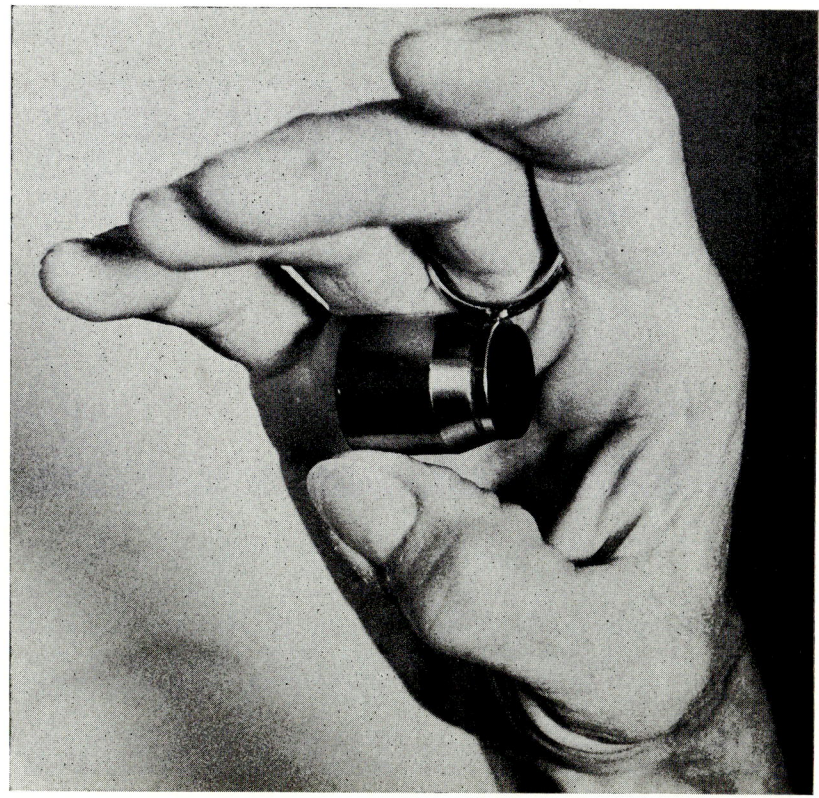

Figure II-3. The ring telescope may be held in the palm of the hand or worn on a neck chain. Young people accept this aid cosmetically.

acceptable. The right-handed patient can wear it on the left hand hold the hand up to the eye, and view the blackboard while taking notes with the right hand. The Keeler ring scope has a 6° field and focuses from infinity to 25 feet; the Hellinger ring scope has a field of 5° and focuses from infinity to 3 feet.

The Selsi 6x-8x prism monocular is focusable. The 6x has a field of 11°, and the 8x has a field of 8°. The 6x objective and 8x objective are easily interchangeable even for the low vision patient and can be used for a wide variety of situations, classroom, ballet, plays, and sports.

Higher power magnifications for distance are necessary either when a person has lower acuity than 20/240 or the distance is greater

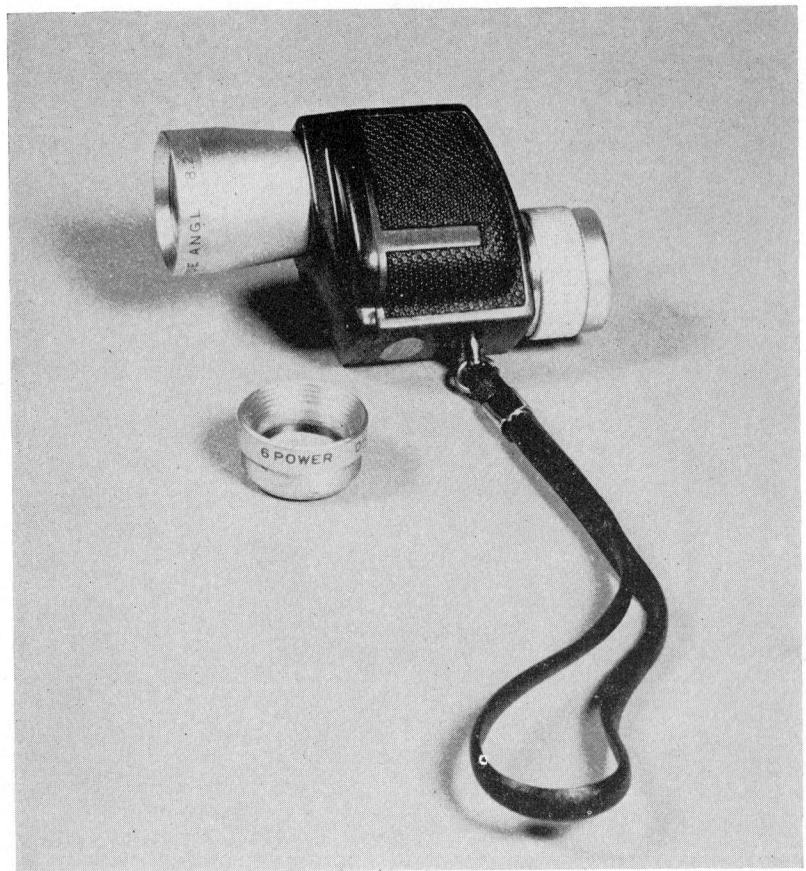

Figure II-4. The Selsi 6x-8x hand telescope is one of the most useful aids. The interchangeable objectives increase the range of use.

than a classroom or small theatre. For large theatres, arenas, and sporting events, binoculars with sufficient magnification can be used. The Selsi 7x to 12x focusable zoom prism monocular with a field varying from 5° to 6° is also an excellent choice for the low vision patient.

However, the 10x focusable Selsi prism mini-monocular which has a 4° field is a poor choice due to the difficulty of object location with this very small field.

CONTACT LENS TELESCOPES: The contact lens telescopic system consists of a plus objective lens in a spectacle frame and a high minus contact lens. The field of view through this system can be as large as

50°; however, the amount of magnification attainable through the system is less than 2x. Because of the mechanical problems of stability of the high minus contact lens and the controlled separation of the ocular and objective lenses, the system has little practical application.

BINOCULARS AND THE SELSI ZOOM: When the residual visual acuity of the low vision patient is very low, or the distance at which he must view is very great, high degrees of magnification are necessary to enable the individual to function. Such magnification is not available in small pocket-size telescopes but is available in binoculars or a large prism monocular.

These low vision aids may be used for viewing:
1. Sports events or theatre.
2. Blackboards.
3. Traffic lights.

The binocular is particularly suited as a low vision aid. The large objective lenses gather light, and thus the image produced by the optical system is enhanced as compared to the image produced by other types of optical systems. Most low vision patients respond to enlargement and image enhancement, and this is the type of image created by binoculars.

A binocular can also be used as both a distance and near system. This works best if the vision in one eye of the low vision patient is much better than the vision in the other eye. In this case the objective lens of the binocular which coincides with the better eye of the patient is used for distance; and a plus cap of sufficient power is placed over the other objective, and that portion of the binocular is used for near objects. When only one objective is being used for distance, the binocular can be better stabilized by resting the binoculars on the superorbital prominence and the side of the nose.

The patient's distance correction can be placed in a lens cap over the ocular lens. Zoom binoculars are available in a 2 to 1 zoom (8x-16x) and are quite advantageous for a person with low vision.

The Selsi prism monocular zoom is available from 7x to 12x. The problem with high powered prism monoculars, especially the zoom type, is that they are large and cumbersome and the individual fatigues when viewing and cannot hold them steady. The Selsi zoom has a place for a stand mount.

TELEMICROSCOPES: A telemicroscope is structurally a Galilean telescope with enough additional plus in the objective lens so that the working distance coincides with the (punctum remotum) front focus of the system.

There is a definite need for low vision near point prescriptions which allow reasonable working distances. A 3x microscopic lens would have a working distance of less than 4 inches. In a particular case it might enable the patient to read, but with such a short working distance it would not allow the person to comfortably write a letter, sign checks, and balance books.

The number of visual tasks requiring a sufficient working distance range from reading music while playing an instrument and playing bridge, to computer programming, filing, and typing.

When the need for an adequate working distance outweighs all other factors, then the telemicroscopic low vision prescription should be considered.

The telemicroscopic prescription differs from the microscopic near point prescription in several ways.

1. The telemicroscope has a greater working distance than a microscope of equal magnification.
2. The telemicroscope has a smaller field of view than a microscope of equal magnification.
3. The telemicroscope has a smaller depth of focus than a microscope of equal magnification.

There are two types of telemicroscopes

1. Any Galilean telescope which has a plus cap placed over the objective lens to focus at the near working distance.
2. A Galilean type telescope which has included in the objective lens sufficient plus to focus at the near working distance.

Keeler Telemicroscopes incorporate the patient's distance Rx in the magnifying units. The units may be mounted in a sturdy spectacle frame or specially mounted in Ary loupe flip-up carriers.* They have a magnification range from 1.6x to 8x. The working distances are standardized. The units are so set in the carrier lens to conform to near point axis.

Oculus Loupe is a telemicroscope which is a pair of spectacles containing the distance Rx and flip-down objectives with an adjust-

---

* Available from Lighthouse Optical Aids Service, 111 E. 59th St., N.Y.C. 10022.

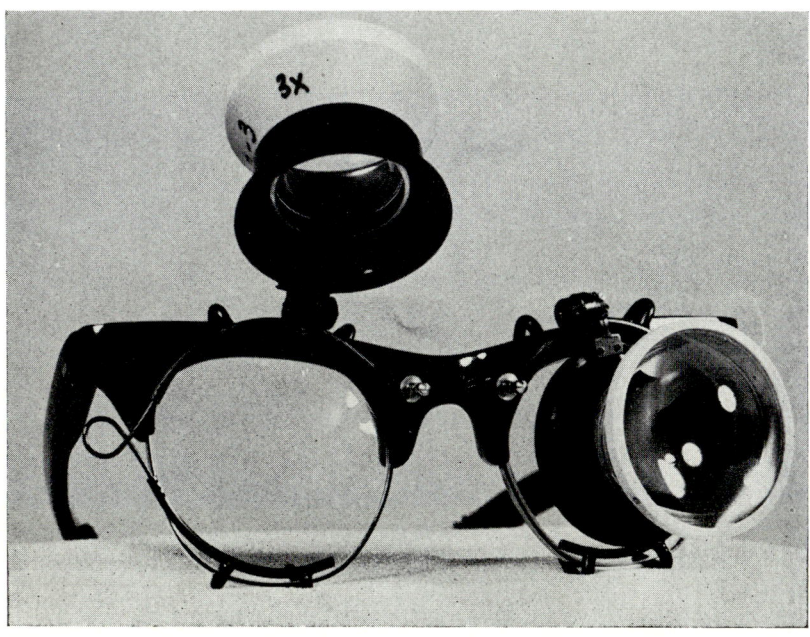

Figure II-5. Telemicroscopes (Keeler) are telescopic units for intermediate and near work. The *add* is incorporated into the objective. They have a standard spectacle mounting but can also be specially mounted in flip-up carriers.

ment for obtaining the near visual axis. The magnification is 1.7x with a 13-inch working distance.

Designs for Vision Telemicroscopes have the patient's distance prescription included in the magnifying units, and the units are placed in the carrier lens so they conform to the near point visual axis. These lenses may be mounted in a sturdy spectacle frame. The magnifications available are 2.5x, 3.5x, and 4x. Any desired working distance can be ordered.

A telemicroscope can also be made using the Designs for Vision distance telescope of either 1.7x, 2.2x, 3x, or 4x and adding a plus cap which snaps on and off. The plus cap is of sufficient power to focus at the desired near working distance.

The practitioner must take extreme care to assure that objectives of the telemicroscope are properly aligned. To obtain the proper alignment the optical axis of the system must coincide with the visual axis of each eye when it is focused on the punctum remotum.

UNUSUAL TYPES OF TELESCOPES: One of the unique uses for the Galilean telescope is its capacity in reverse to widen the environment for someone with severe field loss. Although the patient's field of view becomes wider, the image on the retina is smaller, thus becoming more difficult to discern. This system can only be used if the patient's acuity is between 20/20 and 20/40. Another unusual but seldom used telescopic arrangement is a +3.00 sphere held in front of the uncorrected aphakic eye.

Considerations in Prescribing Telescopes

The most important considerations in prescribing a telescopic system for a low vision patient are as follows
1. Does the lens system fulfill the visual needs of the patient?
2. Will the patient accept the cosmetic appearance of the lens system?

Only a small percentage (approximately 15%) of low vision patients have a need for a telescopic prescription. These patients generally fall into three categories:
1. Students.
2. Driver's licensing candidates.
3. Low vision patients with specific occupational and recreational demands.

In these three types of cases, the visual acuity of the patient is usually no better than 20/70 nor worse than 20/300.

1. *Students.*

In the early classroom years, the student usually goes up to the board to copy homework assignments. In high school and college this is often impossible, and the student must read the black board from his seat. Often a professor will hurriedly work a problem on the board as a form of explanation. Thus, the student with low vision needs help at this distance in order to follow board work in the classroom.

2. *Driver's Licensing.*

Several states have programs to license candidates with low vision, who wear Bioptic telescopic lenses. This allows the people to have the mobility necessary for equal occupational opportunities. In most areas

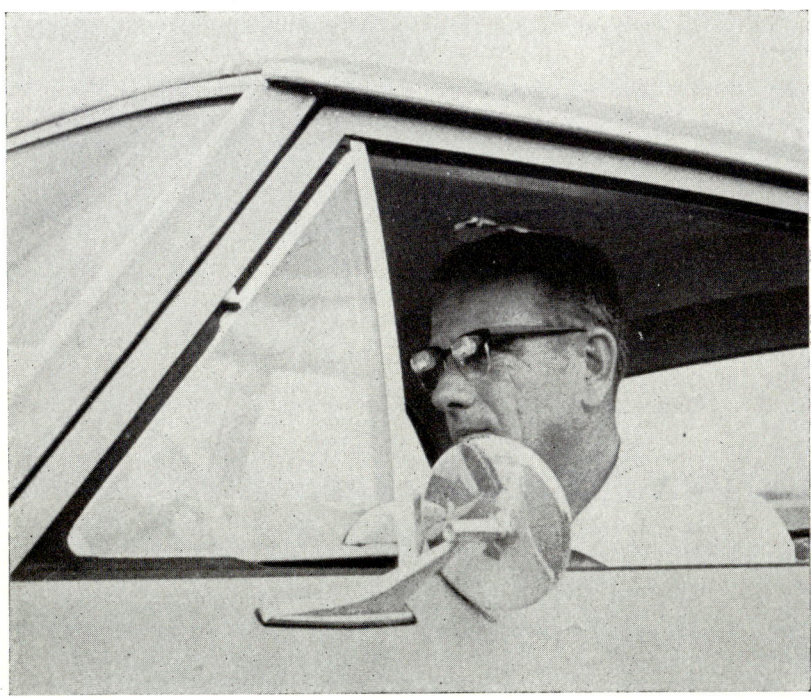

Figure II-6. A licensed driver wearing 2.2x Bioptic I telescopes set high in the lens carrier to allow good peripheral vision. Spotting through the telescopic unit requires a quick movement of the eyes, much as one would use to see objects in a rearview mirror.

of this country a car is not a luxury but a necessity because there is little or no public transportation. A car is necessary not only to have a good job but also sometimes to have any job. In rural communities a car is the only means of traveling to nearby towns.

3. *Occupational and Recreational Needs.*

Occasionally an occupation requires an individual to see at a distance from a fixed position or to see at an intermediate distance such as 30 inches for playing music or typing. In such cases a telescope with a reading cap or telemicroscope would be appropriate.

Many recreational interests require good distance vision; horse racing, football, ballet, plays. These visual demands can be fulfilled by binoculars and opera glasses of sufficient magnification to enable the patient to enjoy the event.

As stated earlier, a most important consideration in prescribing telescopes is cosmetic acceptance or rejection. The use of any telescope, a Bioptic or hand held telescope, is an admission to the world that one has a severe visual handicap. It is the unusual low vision patient who is willing to demonstrate that he has a visual loss.

Most students will wear Bioptic lenses when seated in the classroom but will put them away when changing classes. A young girl may use them to see the blackboard when she is ten or twelve years old but may stop wearing them when she is fifteen and the boys are watching.

Summary

Although telescopic prescriptions do not have wide spread application for low vision patients, there are certain situations in which these prescriptions increase the ability of the patient to use his residual vision.

· CHAPTER III ·
Treating Subnormal Vision In Aphakia

CHARLES R. MOORE

ALL OF us at one time or another have been frustrated by a patient who has become increasingly unhappy with the world of aphakic vision which is now complicated by subnormal vision. This could happen either to a patient who had only recently experienced a technically perfect cataract operation but was subsequently found to have unsuspected macular pathology, or to one who developed macular problems many years after a successful cataract operation.

What happens to the average aphakic patient whose vision seems to be less than perfect? Does the busy practitioner see his problem for what it really is? We cannot always evaluate the visual result until we have tried our best to provide every patient with the most efficient refraction we can.

It is absolutely impossible to tell how efficiently any given patient can function in the world of aphakia unless he is wearing the best aphakic refraction that can be prescribed. All of us are familiar with the many technical problems with aphakic refractions that cause a patient to see only 20/40 or 20/50 with his permanent spectacles even though he could be refracted in the office to 20/20. This is not desirable, but most patients learn to live with it. However, when the best refracted acuity is near 20/80 and the patient still loses two or three more lines due to an inaccurate translation of the refraction into glasses, we then have an unnecessarily handicapped patient. Most of these technical problems can now be overcome by using the "Zero Error" *Aphakic Refracting Kit* designed by Dr. Robert C. Welsh.[1,2] The kit contains six pairs of thin, +11.00 aspheric lenses mounted in permanent frames, set at the more commonly used pupillary distances, and styled for both men and women. For the

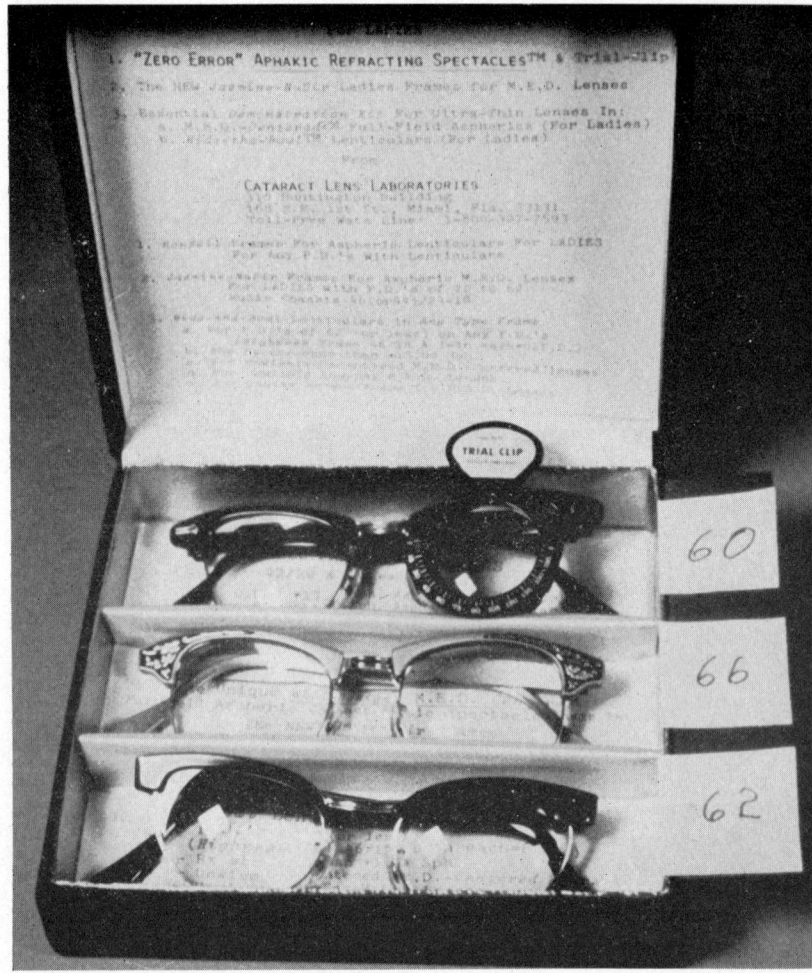

Figure III-1. Three aphakic spectacles styled for women in the Aphakic Refracting Kit. Having + 11.00, thin, aspheric lenses premounted in frames simplifies refraction of aphakic patients. Over-refraction is performed using the Halberg clip.

refraction, place the permanent frame with the correct P.D. on the individual patient and perform a standard trial lens over-refraction with the Halberg trial lens clip or phoropter. This abolishes the need for a distometer (and thus vertex errors which can be as great as 1.75 diopters). It avoids up to 0.75 diopters of error possible when shifting from either spheric trial lenses or very steep and thicker temporaries to permanent ultrathin and flatter lenses of equal power. Because the exact center of the lens is in line with the patient's visual axis, one avoids up to 1.25 diopters of error that can occur if the patient is looking eccentrically through a trial lens, a temporary spectacle lens, or especially a phoropter lens. It also prevents up to 0.87 diopters of error due to improper pantoscopic tilt duplication. Excessive pantoscopic tilt (over 5°) leads to cylindrical errors at 180° axis. If no cylinder is present, it creates one at axis 180°, and in cases where a cylinder is present, it deviates it towards axis 180°. It is extremely important during this over-refraction to remind the patient not to tilt or turn the head in an attempt to clear the vision and therefore create an error in the final prescription. By thus having a final prescription adjusted very close and low with an accurate P.D., we have a uniform way of obtaining maximal visual efficiency from every aphakic prescription, therefore avoiding the frustration of regrinds and changes. Another advantage provided by this kit is that one can now order *minimal effective diameter* centered lenses (rather than the standard lenticular lens) for at least 90 percent of the patients.[2] These superior lenses are both a great improvement functionally and cosmetically. Prior to this, all of the author's attempts to order plastic, full field aspheric lenses with *minimal effective diameter* centering from other companies had been utter disasters.

The basis for fitting *minimal effective diameter* lenses is in choosing a frame with a small vertical vs horizontal difference, (i.e. Ronsir Shuron Continental is a 6-difference shape), and controlling the horizontal eye and bridge size to match as closely as possible the distance P.D..

Example:
Patient Distance P.D.	64
Frame 44/20	64
46/18	64

As one can see, strong plus lenses require little if any decentration, and the edge thickness can be controlled laterally in this manner. Of course edge thickness top and bottom will be controlled by the shape difference. Ideally an M.E.D. grind would be most effective in a perfectly round shape if spherical or ovoid if cylinderical with a multitude of eye and bridge sizes to *tailor* the frame to the patient's exact facial measurements.

It is also of interest to note that, unlike most conventional grinding whose base curves both match regardless of powers, M.E.D. blanks are chosen which will result in inside curves of 1 diopter or less. This technique helps to reduce the bulbous appearances of cataract glasses and decreases the magnification.

By using "new M.E.D." techniques of nasal decentration and after choosing the correctly fitted frame, a significant number of people can gain temporal field and have a 46-size eyepiece provide the vision normally obtained from a size 50 eyepiece.

It is extremely important for many aphakics especially those who have subnormal visual problems to have two pairs of permanent spectacles. By using full field aspheric M.E.D. lenses with no bifocal added, the patient can gain an inferior-temporal field of vision and have no distortion when he looks down stairs or steps off curbs. He can use these glasses at all times except when he wants to read or work up close for sustained periods of time. He can be taught to slide his single vision spectacles down his nose until he gains the needed magnification or use Magna Adds® when distance Rx is less than +12.00. In my experience a vast majority of patients prefer this system if they are properly educated to its advantages, and they definitely travel with more grace and skill. Medicare will pay for two sets of permanent spectacles if the practitioner will specify that one is for distance and one is for reading. It is always a good idea to remind patients with subnormal vision that proper lighting while reading can make the difference in success and failure. Because of the need for strong light, however, the practitioner should avoid excessive amount of tint in most aphakic spectacles for the partially sighted.

Let us say that we now have a well-motivated patient and all of the technical problems of aphakic refractions worked out, but he still can not read. There are a number of good hand or stand magnifiers available in the New York Lighthouse Magnifier Kit[3] that are well accepted by patients and the ideal starting place for a patient who wants to learn how to use magnification. Unfortunately, if we go much over a 3.50 diopter or 4.00 diopter add, we lose binocularity in aphakia because of the increased convergence requirements. As a rule of thumb, with a vision of 20/50, a +4.00 add is needed to read J5 print, 20/100 requires +8.00, and 20/200 requires +16.00. The American Optical Company[4] has three standard (+6.00, +12.00, +18.00) bifocal segments which can be incorporated into any aphakic prescription in an Aolite® lens for a minimal increase in cost to the patient. Naturally all of these involve only monocular reading but are readily available. Another near-aid is the Press-on Optics® D-25 segs which have base-in Fresnel prism built into the adds and are mounted in trial lenses for use with a trial frame or Halberg® clip. Also useful in this area are the Magna Add Clip-over lenses which allow a temporary boost in magnification and can be removed after use. They come in three powers of +1.50 diopters, +2.25, and +3.00 diopters.

If a patient must have better distance vision, the means of correction are very limited, but a hand held Selsi 6x-8x telescope[5] is one of the most popular items. The Designs for Vision Bioptic spectacles can incorporate a telescope for distance and a microscopic button for near objects on the same spectacle lens. The major drawback to these is that they require a sophisticated practitioner to prescribe them and a patient who has a sophisticated need for this use of magnification. The severely handicapped aphakic patient (20/100 or worse with best corrected vision) has a special problem with distance vision that can best be solved by the use of either hard or soft contact lenses. By successfully fitting these patients with a contact lens, we may not improve their distance vision at all, but we return them to a more *phakic type* visual field with the contact lens. This allows us to use one of the most successful binocular phakic aids which is the American Optical half frame which incorporates base-in prism.[4] For the monocular patients, the contact lens provides a less magnified image. I urge anyone who has not tried this idea to do so, and I think my enthusiasm will be shared.

REFERENCES

1. Welsh, Robert C.: *Postoperative-Cataract Spectacle Lenses.* Miami, Miami Educational Press, 1961.
2. Welsh, Robert C.: *Aphakic Spectacle Dispensing Guide.* Miami, Cataract Lens Laboratories Inc.

3. The New York Association for the Blind: Lighthouse Low Vision Aid Kit. Lighthouse Low Vision Service, New York.
4. American Optical Company, Southbridge.
5. Lighthouse Low Vision Service: *Catalogue of Optical Aids*, 3rd ed., New York, Lighthouse Low Vision Service, 1973.
6. Designs for Vision, New York.

· CHAPTER IV ·
Closed Circuit Television: Its Value In Low Vision

Morris J. Mintz

Introduction

THE TIME has come to clear the smoke surrounding the value of closed circuit television (CCTV) magnification and place it in proper perspective

Magnification has long been known as an aid for low vision. The optical principles of visual aids were spelled out over fifty years ago and summarized by Stein and Gradle[1] in 1924. Any changes since then have been refinements in design, such as aspheric surfaces, and more cosmetically acceptable units.

With the advent of CCTV, a new dimension was added to magnification electronic enhancement. It is, however, only another visual aid in our armamentarium as Davis, Asarkof, and Tallman[2] recently pointed out so well. It can be considered a further extension of a refraction.

The advantages of the CCTV over conventional optical visual aids are:
1. Magnification is obtained electronically as well as optically.
2. Viewing can be accomplished at a comfortable distance from the screen as compared to the close viewing distance required by optical magnification.
3. Magnification can be varied at will with minimal adjustments.
4. Contrast of image on background can be intensified.
5. Brightness is adjustable.
6. A negative image (reversal) of printed material can be easily obtained, e.g. white on black from black on white.
7. There is less aberration with electronic magnification than with optical aids.

8. No special training is required in its use other than simple technical skills needed to operate the equipment.

The basic components of a CCTV are:
1. Monitor.
2. Television camera.
3. Zoom lens preferably, although a fixed focus lens can be used for a fixed magnification.
4. A source of bright, even light.
5. A stand for mounting the components, including the monitor.

Variations in the type of mounting-stand and configuration of the components can make each complete unit more easily adaptable in use. Among these options are a moveable X-Y table, a scanning device, a camera which can be tilted from vertical to horizontal, and a mirror device so that the camera can be mounted below the monitor.

Early development of the CCTV reader was delayed by its high initial cost. Reduction of costs, especially the camera, made a CCTV unit for the partially sighted practical. Potts and Volk[3] first described such a reading aid in 1959 although others were working on similar devices at the time. Genensky[4] in 1970 described a practical model which later was modified and produced commercially. There have been further changes in the CCTV units, all in the interest of reduced costs, reduced size and weight, increased portability, and increased convenience of use.

Some type of CCTV should be available in every low vision clinic. Its primary use would be in reassuring patients that they can still read ordinary print when it is magnified. Whenever we see a patient for the first time, especially an older individual with a recent visual loss, we demonstrate to him with the CCTV that he still has enough vision to read. Then we return to trials of the various optical aids that he will more readily accept.

Rehabilitation is probably the most valuable use of the CCTV. We can consider rehabilitation in its broadest sense, social, educational, and vocational. At the social level it can be very important for an individual to be able to read his own mail or to spend a few minutes a day reading portions of the daily newspaper. Motivation is the most important factor in acceptance and use of the CCTV and educational background a close second. One who has always read will use it: one who has read little will not use it.

Case Histories

P.B. is an eighty-four-year-old male with macular degeneration and corrected visual acuity 2/300 in each eye. He has had a CCTV for four years. He uses it four hours per day but fatigues after reading a newspaper for twenty minutes.

A CCTV was placed in the Kalamazoo Central Library by the local Lions Club. It was to be used by the geriatric partially sighted population in the area. The librarian informed us that after the first few months there were no requests to use the instrument. Shall we assume that the inconvenience of going to the library was too great or that motivation was too little, or is it a combination of both? Or did they prefer simpler aids?

L.L. is a twenty-five-year-old female with retrolental fibroplasia and corrected visual acuity 10/200-10/400. With optical aids she can read only magazine print. With the CCTV she can read any size print easily. She has used a CCTV for over three years while working as a computer programmer. She would occasionally go to work early to do some personal reading. She has now purchased a CCTV for her personal use at home.

G.P. is a thirty-four-year-old male with bilateral microcornea and corrected visual acuity 10/300 in the right eye only. With optical aids he reads very slowly "with his nose." He can read easily with the CCTV and uses it while he works as a computer programmer for the Internal Revenue Service.

J.W. is a forty-five-year-old male with optic atrophy secondary to late diabetes and pituitary stalk section, and corrected visual acuity 10/400. He has retained his job with one of the large auto companies because he can read a printout for production scheduling with the CCTV. He is at a managerial level of employment, and his experience is much more valuable than his sight, although being able to see the printed numbers certainly gives him more confidence in making decisions.

H.C. is a twenty-four-year-old female with retrolental fibroplasia and corrected visual acuity 10/160 in her only eye. She can read with an 8x spectacle aid but finds in her work as a medical records librarian that the CCTV is indispensable in using the medical dictionary and in reading the text in charts. The latter is probably due to the illiterate scribbling that most of us physicians employ in our notes.

K.J. is a twenty-six-year-old female with atypical retinitis pigmentosa and nystagmus and corrected visual acuity of O.D. 10/150 and O.S. 10/100. With visual aids she can read newsprint very slowly, but with black on white on the CCTV she can read more easily and faster. She is employed as a secretary and receptionist.

D.K. is a thirty-year-old male with retinitis pigmentosa and posterior polar cataracts. Visual acuity is "moving objects," but, when the pupils are dilated, corrected visual acuity is 10/400 O.U.. The visual field is very constricted. He is a social worker and used Braille exclusively. He would occasionally use a 20x hand loupe to help him read very laboriously a name on a form. With the CCTV he is now able to fill out his own case reports and to read his correspondence. He prefers using a 12-inch monitor but can use the larger screen as well.

A.T. is a forty-four-year-old male with progressive optic atrophy, corrected visual acuity 10/40 in each eye, and he can read with +7.00 adds. He is a music teacher and finds that the CCTV is the only device that can help him read his music conveniently while he is teaching. He moves his music manually under the camera and finds it not too inconvenient.

We feel that the educational area has not been explored sufficiently using the CCTV. We have seen children just being taught to read who have a corrected visual acuity in the range of 10/200 to 10/400. They were being taught to read "with their nose" and were making headway, but the extra ease of both teaching and reading with CCTV was beyond description. Red tape and economic factors often prevented a CCTV being made available to these children.

P.N. is a fifteen-year-old female with congenital glaucoma, nystagmus, and very scarred corneas. Her visual acuity is light perception in the right eye and 1/700 in the left eye. She had been using Braille and carried her book with her when she appeared for her first examination. Her mother had taught her print reading using very large print. She is able to read standard print with the CCTV, but it took almost a year of unwinding red tape to obtain one for her. Even though her prognosis is guarded for retaining vision, she at present can be more efficient in obtaining her education.

K.G. is a fourteen-year-old male with congenital optic atrophy with nystagmus and with corrected visual acuity O.D. 10/150, O.S. 10/200. He was educated in Braille. 4x miniature telescopes mounted on glasses give him equivalent visual acuity of 20/30 and 20/70. The +12.00 caps for the telescopes allow him to read, but the field is too restricted. This boy is a child prodigy on the piano. He played the church organ at the age of three. He was taught the piano without reading music. He could immediately play any tune that was hummed to him. He now uses the CCTV to read music that he has not heard. He reads a bar or two at a time, plays the music, and commits it to memory. The CCTV is alongside the piano.

Summary

The CCTV is another visual aid for the partially sighted which should be available in every low vision clinic. It can extend the ability to read where optical aids fail. It can make reading more convenient and practical in certain situations for education and vocational rehabilitation.

REFERENCES

1. Stein, J. C., and Gradle, H.: Telescopic spectacles and magnifiers as aids to poor vision, 1924, reprint ed., *Trans Am Acad Ophthalmol Otolaryngol,* 77:229-253, 1973.
2. Davis, P., Asarkof, J., and Tallman, C. B.: A closed circuit television system as a reading aid for visually handicapped persons. *The New Outlook for the Blind,* 67:97-01, 1973.
3. Potts, A. M., Volk, D., and West, S. S.: A television reader as a subnormal vision aid. *Am J Ophthalmol,* 47:4, 1959.
4. Genensky, Samuel M.: *Closed Circuit Television and the Education of the Partially Sighted.* Santa Monica, The Rand Corporation, 1970.

· CHAPTER V ·
Nonoptical Aids

CLARE M. HOOD

WHEN A patient first comes to a low vision clinic, his expectation based on his experience as a normally sighted person is that glasses will correct his problems.

His earliest disappointment is to discover that glasses may help him for reading and close work but are cumbersome and restrictive for many of his daily nonreading activities.

If one asks the average sighted-person what he considers the most important visual activity, he would say reading. If one asks a partially sighted person the same question, he might say that reading is not as important as other simple, daily physical tasks. We do not consider how much of a day is spent in visual activities other than reading, nor do we give much consideration to the existence of people who never did enjoy reading.

It is estimated that for 30 percent of a patient's activities an optical device is not as effective as a nonoptical device. These nonoptical aids are not lenses nor do they contain lenses. They are devices which allow residual vision to be used in such a way that the person feels he is more normal. These nonoptical aids must function as a supplement to optical aids and are prescribed, as a rule, after optical aids have been thoroughly explored. Only after the patient has realized the limitations of aids can he express his other needs to the examiner or assistants.

The nonoptical aids discussed in this chapter are the ones most frequently used by low vision patients.

Lighting

Correct lighting is probably the most important nonoptical aid. There is no formula for predicting the placement or intensity of a light

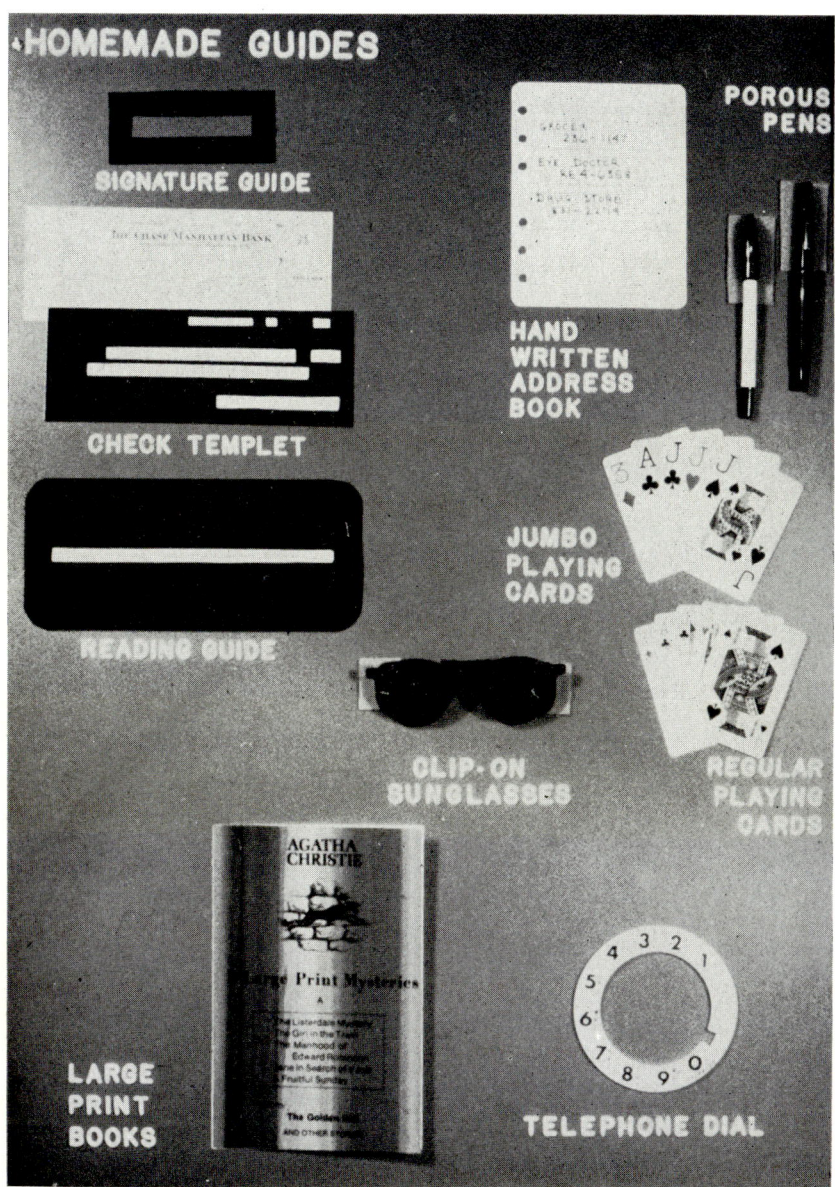

Figure V-1. Common nonoptical aids.

source needed for any given patient. As a rule, the light source should be in front of the patient's face and as close to the page as possible. This arrangement gives maximum intensity without glare. The lamp chosen should have a flexible, adjustable arm. A correct light source if often as effective as a stronger prescription. A lamp should have a solid base to prevent tipping when used by the older patient. Lamps should use standard incandescent bulbs or fluorescent tubes because of cost and availability.

Writing Aids

Writing with a strong optical aid is difficult because the focal distance is too short to allow a pen or pencil to be held comfortably. There are nonoptical writing devices that patients can use with their regular glasses which allow them to maintain a more normal writing distance.

Porous Tip Pens

A nylon-tipped pen with black ink for maximum contrast can be used to print letters large enough to be seen by the patient. He can write and read back what he has written. Family and friends should be encouraged to carry on their correspondence using these pens and writing or printing clearly.

Special Writing Paper

Partially sighted older patients are embarrassed to send a letter with crooked lines. Bold Ruled Paper[1] is special white paper lined in black at 7/16-inch intervals. Although lined paper is most often used by school children, older patients like to place a sheet of bold ruled paper under air mail or translucent stationary as a guide. However, many adult patients prefer using their own stationery and one of the line guides.

Line Guides

The Script Writing Board is a plastic board either 3 inches by 5 inches or 5 inches by 8 inches with raised lines. Stationery is placed over the board and the person writes within the raised lines. Practical patients have often discovered that a 3 inch-by 5 inch-index card held under the line is the simplest homemade guide. Script Signature Guides are smaller than writing boards and are available in metal or cardboard with one single line for signatures.

Typewriters

Since writing legibly and comfortably is always a chore for people wearing low vision lenses, typing is a logical communication skill to be suggested.

Learning to type may present a welcome challenge for the partially sighted person who is trying to find new interests or continue his current occupation. A few companies which manufacture typewriters show models of larger type size in their catalogues.

Typing should be started as early as possible for all partially sighted children. Their school work is more presentable and legible. Typing is also an excellent skill for schoolage children who have problems in motor coordination and who have poor handwriting.

Check Guides[1,2]

Keeping patients independent means privacy in financial matters. A slotted guide made to fit a patient's individual check and stub is essential. These can be either commercially produced or homemade.[1]

Telephone Dials

For the standard nonpushbutton phone, two types of dials are available.[1] One type has enlarged white letters and numbers on a black background. Clinical preference has been for a white base with black numbers which are either embossed or flat. To date, patients with macular disease with or without aphakia have chosen the nonembossed type. Some local telephone companies may provide dials with large numbers. People who have pushbutton phones have discovered that darkening the number with a marking pen eliminates difficulty in seeing.

Sewing Aids

Patients like to continue their customary activities. Sewing is both a necessity and a pleasure.

For hand sewing, any needle can be stabilized for threading by sticking it into a cork. The cork is then held in the hand and can be more easily moved into the best near focus either by using an aid or bright illumination.

Self-Threading Needles

These needles have a spring notch in the top of the eye of the needle. The thread is stretched across the notch and pulled down into the eye. The use of needle threaders is also familiar to patients who may have used them prior to their vision problem.

Large Print Tape Measures

A large print tape measure with ¾-inch numbers is useful for many things besides sewing, for example, carpentry, tile laying and cabinet installation. Older people have lifelong skills and interests which can be maintained with such simple devices.

Playing Cards

Large print playing cards allow many patients for whom card playing is an important recreation, to scan their hand at a normal distance and see the cards on the table. Large print playing cards are standard size cards with enlarged numbers and symbols which are not objectionable to normally sighted players. Bridge or pinochle decks are available.

Visorettes

Some patients are bothered by light but cannot tolerate absorptive lenses because they reduce visual acuity. Yet glare itself is another factor in reducing vision especially in macular degeneration and cortical lens opacities. For these patients a plastic visor attached to a spectacle frame blocks overhead glare.[1]

Reading Stands

Patients who cannot hold a book because of physical disability, can be helped by using a reading stand. Stands are available in most department stores and mail order catalogues.

Music students and secretaries use stands raised to eye level for their work. The Gore stand[1] and the Shafer stand[1] are made especially for this purpose.

Aids for Diabetics

Diabetics with eye involvement provide a significant patient load for most low vision clinics. Because of the variable nature of their visual acuity they cannot rely solely on optical aids to manage their medication regime.

Available on prescription from the American Foundation for the Blind are several types of insulin syringes and needle guides. A description of nondisposable set syringes[2] follows.

1. Becton-Dickinson Company produces a short-barrel insulin syringe with an adjustable screw stop which regulates dosage on an 80-unit scale (this may be changed to 100 units).
2. Hill Accurate Dosage Insulin Syringe is a long-barrel 80-unit scale with metal plunger and double ring lock. When the correct dosage is drawn, the rings click. This signal can be heard and felt by the patient. This syringe is the easiest to set and to use.
3. The European syringe is a complicated system which is the only syringe available for the diabetic who has to take varying doses. The dosage is calibrated by a system of audible clicks, each representing ¼ cc. The patient must be carefully instructed and he must have a good memory.

Needle Guides

Many patients have difficulty getting the needle into the rubber seal on top of the insulin bottle.

1. A funnel-shaped aluminum cap which fits over the top of the Eli Lilly insulin vial guides the needle to the center of the seal. It can be left on the bottle for identification of the vial being used and wiped prior to use with an antiseptic sponge.
2. A notched aluminum guide is an older device which is still available. The needle is placed in the "V" and the vial pushed sideways towards the needle. Most patients seem to find this device awkward to use.

Large Print

Having to hold regular-sized print close to the spectacle aid is tiring for some patients, especially if they have a respiratory problem or limitation of joint movements. Since enlarged print can be seen farther away, the strength of the optical aid can be reduced to get the patient a few more inches away from his reading. Other patients who have severe vision limitations may not be able to read regular print easily with a strong optical aid. If they do not have access to a closed circuit television, large print read with a strong plus lens may provide their only contact with printed material.

Large print is not only a matter of personal preference. It may be a necessity in some cases. Large print books for adults are available from most libraries. Information can be obtained from the library of The New York Association for the Blind and from the National Association for the Visually Handicapped in New York. *The New York Times* and newly designed *Reader's Digest* are obtained from their source.

Talking Books should be mentioned as a supplement to other resources. Even when patients can read well with an optical aid, they may prefer to listen to books on tapes or records particularly if they were rapid readers before their visual impairment. Local libraries supply an application blank for obtaining the books and recording machines.

Once they understand the limitation of lenses resourceful patients tend to use their own initiative in suggesting or finding supplementary nonoptical aids. Patients who are not resourceful, who are depressed, or who lack initative need skilled supportive instruction and training to solve problems intensified by loss of sight. In summary, remember to think of nonoptical aids for the low vision patient.

REFERENCES

1. *Catalogue of Optical Aids.* 3rd ed. rev. New York, New York Lighthouse Low Vision Service, 1973.
2. *Aids and Appliances*, 19th ed., *American Foundation for the Blind,* New York, 1973-1974.

· SECTION TWO ·
Development of Visual Aids

CHAPTER VI

The Optical Design of Spectacle Magnifiers

Donald B. Whitney

ONE OF the most common optical aids used in low vision applications is the spectacle magnifier. It offers the patient magnifications of up to ten times and more and leaves the hands free to manipulate the reading material. Such aids are usually lightweight, portable, and relatively inexpensive.

Two of the more serious drawbacks to spectacle magnifiers are their rather short working distances and their limited fields of view. The first often requires the reading material to be held so close that adequate lighting presents a problem. The second allows the patient to see only a few letters at a time, thereby making the reading task a difficult and tedious one.

The question naturally arises Why not design lenses with greater working distances and larger fields of view? Clearly, this is the task ahead of us, but it is not a simple one. I would like to discuss briefly some of the optical principles involved in the hope that a better understanding of these principles will shed some light on what the future may hold.

When we define an ophthalmic lens in terms of its dioptric power, we are normally referring to its Effective Power. This is the reciprocal of its back focus (distance between the rear surface of the lens and its focal point) expressed in meters.

This is what we measure on a Lensometer. Note that there is parallel light on the object side of the lens, and the situation is one in which light is coming from a distant object.

It makes sense, when one thinks about it, to be concerned with the *location* of the image relative to the lens vertex. After all, in a normal corrective situation the problem is one of image location: we want the image to fall on the retina.

[51]

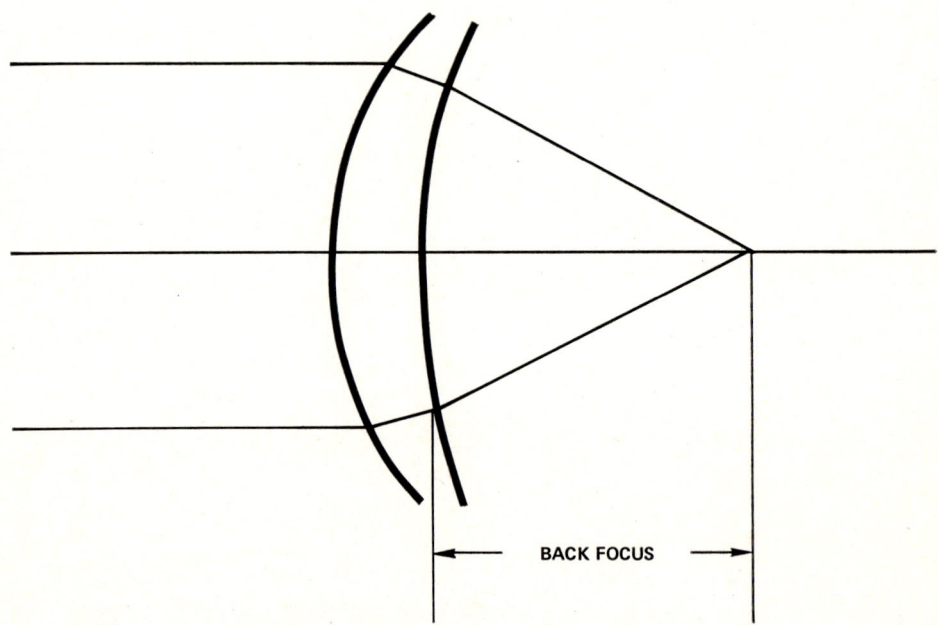

Figure VI-1. The Dioptric Power (effective power) of a lens is the reciprocal of its Back Focus expressed in meters.

The spectacle magnifier represents a somewhat different situation. In the first place, light is coming from a near object and is thus diverging as it enters the front surface. For a relaxed (unaccommodated) eye, parallel light emerges from the ocular surface.

However, a more important difference is that the role of a magnifier is to increase image *size*, and image size is dependent on Equivalent Power, not Effective Power. Let us see what that means.

Consider, for a moment, a lens or lens system as a black box. Assume that the black box represents a well-corrected lens system, and assume that parallel light entering one side of the box emerges from the other side and comes to a focus. If we now extend these rays so that they intersect, the point of intersection lies on what we

The Optical Design of Spectacle Magnifiers 53

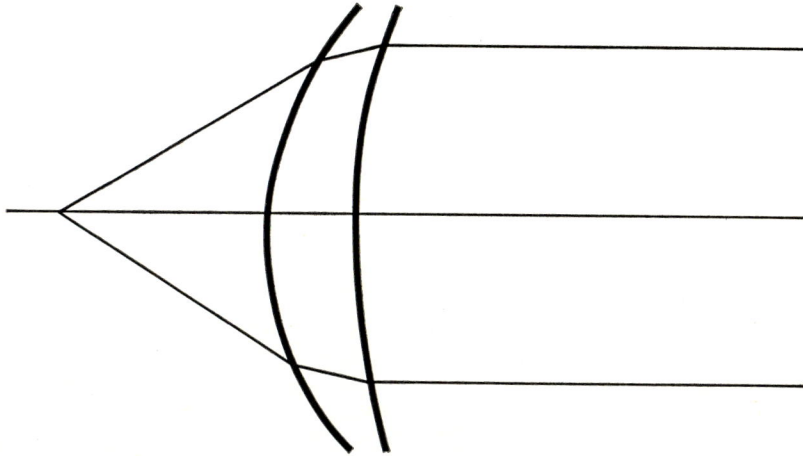

Figure VI-2. Light coming from a near object through a spectacle magnifier.

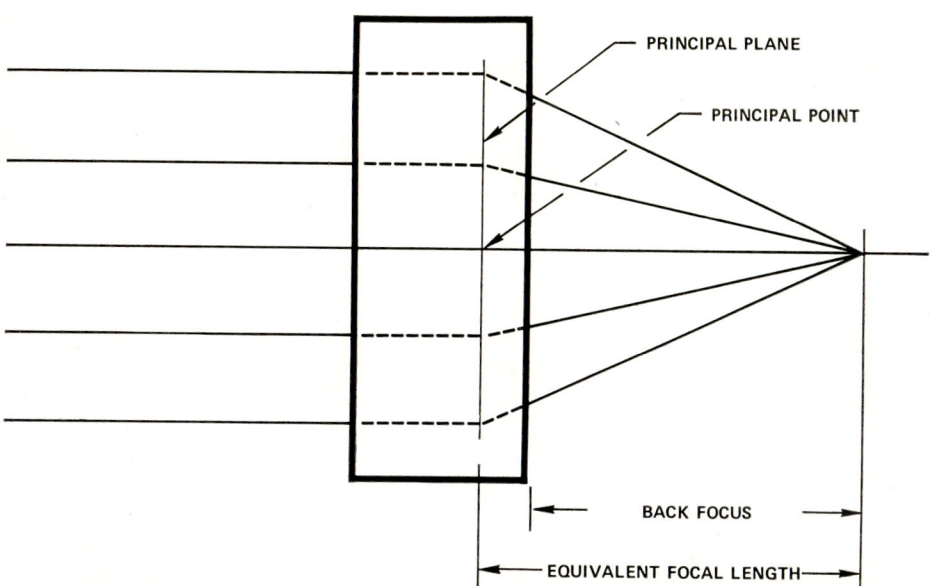

Figure VI-3. Equivalent Focal Length and Back Focus are rarely the same.

call the second principal plane. By introducing additional rays, we further define that plane, and the spot where it intersects the axis we call the second principal point. The distance between this second principal point and the focal point is called the Equivalent Focal Length. Since the second principal point seldom falls on the rear surface of the lens, Equivalent Focal Length and Back Focus are rarely the same.

$$\text{EFFECTIVE POWER (DIOPTERS)} = \frac{1}{\text{BACK FOCUS (Meters)}}$$

$$\text{EQUIVALENT POWER (DIOPTERS)} = \frac{1}{\text{EQUIVALENT FOCAL LENGTH (Meters)}}$$

Figure VI-4. The Equivalent Power as the reciprocal of the Equivalent Focal Length determines the power of a spectacle magnifier.

Earlier we defined Effective Power (or the dioptric power as measured on a Lensometer), as the reciprocal of the Back Focus. Equivalent Power, a term not defined previously, is the reciprocal of the Equivalent Focal Length. This is what determines the power of a spectacle magnifier.

The numbering system used in identifying magnifying power is based on the assumption that the unaided eye can see comfortably at a reading distance of 25 cms (10 inches). Thus, a lens having an Equivalent Focal Length of 25 cms is considered to have a magnifying power of unity (1x). Such a lens has an Equivalent Power of 4 diopters.

$$\text{EQUIVALENT POWER} = \frac{1}{25 \text{ cm}} = \frac{1}{.25 \text{ meters}} = 4 \text{ DIOPTERS}$$

Figure VI-5. A lens with an Equivalent Power of 4 diopters is considered to have a magnifying power of unity (1x).

A lens having an Equivalent Focal Length of 2.5 cms would have an Equivalent Power of 40 diopters. Since it would enable the patient to hold his reading material ten times as close, 2.5 cms (1 inch), such a lens would be marked 10x.

The relationships among Equivalent Focal Length, Equivalent Power, and Magnifying Power are shown in the following table.

TABLE VI-I

RELATIONSHIPS AMONG EQUIVALENT FOCAL LENGTH, EQUIVALENT POWER, AND MAGNIFYING POWER

Equivalent Focal Length		Equivalent Power	Magnifying Power
12.5 cm	4.0 in	8 Diopters	2x
6.2	2.5	16	4x
4.2	1.7	24	6x
3.1	1.2	32	8x
2.5	1.0	40	10x
2.1	0.8	48	12x

It can be seen that Magnifying Power is simply the Equivalent Power divided by 4.

$$\text{MAGNIFYING POWER (x)} = \frac{\text{EQUIVALENT POWER (DIOPTERS)}}{4}$$

Figure VI-6. The Magnifying Power of a lens is the Equivalent Power divided by 4.

It is important to note that it is Equivalent Power, not Effective Power (Lensometer Power), which is used in this equation. The two are not the same, and so it follows that Magnifying Power cannot be determined by lensometer measurement. Approximations can be made by dividing the Lensometer Powers by 4; but it must be recognized that such an approach has built-in errors, and these errors are often quite significant in the high-powered lenses used in low vision. The errors may become gross if two or more lenses are combined.

Let us look at some examples. We will work with plastic lenses all having Lensometer Powers of +40.00 diopters and center thicknesses of 12 mm.

The example in Figure VI-9 is interesting; it is a special case in which the Lensometer Power and the Equivalent Power are the same.

In spectacle magnifier application, parallel light will emerge from the ocular side of the lens by assuming a relaxed (unaccommodated) eye. Thus, if we make the lens planoconvex and position the lens

EQUICONVEX

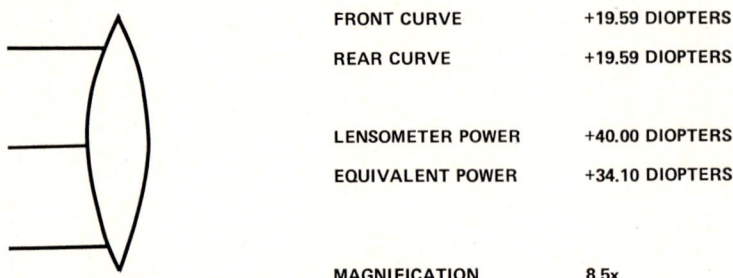

FRONT CURVE	+19.59 DIOPTERS
REAR CURVE	+19.59 DIOPTERS
LENSOMETER POWER	+40.00 DIOPTERS
EQUIVALENT POWER	+34.10 DIOPTERS
MAGNIFICATION	8.5x

Figure VI-7. The equiconvex lens has a Lensometer Power of +40 D and and Equivalent Power of only +34.1 D.

PLANOCONVEX

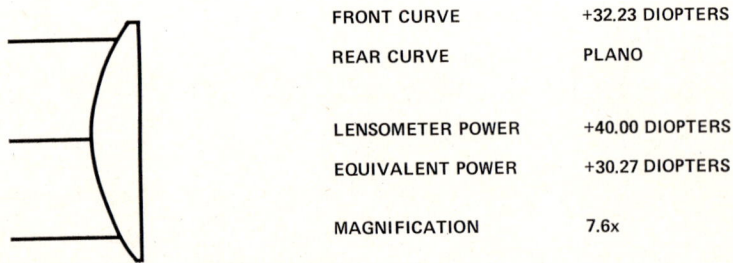

FRONT CURVE	+32.23 DIOPTERS
REAR CURVE	PLANO
LENSOMETER POWER	+40.00 DIOPTERS
EQUIVALENT POWER	+30.27 DIOPTERS
MAGNIFICATION	7.6x

Figure VI-8. The planoconvex lens has a Lensometer Power of +40 D and an Equivalent Power of only +30.2 D.

PLANOCONVEX (REVERSED)

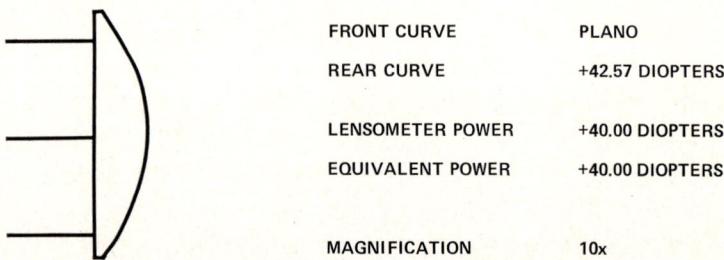

FRONT CURVE	PLANO
REAR CURVE	+42.57 DIOPTERS
LENSOMETER POWER	+40.00 DIOPTERS
EQUIVALENT POWER	+40.00 DIOPTERS
MAGNIFICATION	10x

Figure VI-9. The reversed planoconvex lens has a Lensometer Power of +40 D and an Equivalent Power of +40 D. The magnification equals the Lensometer Power.

The Optical Design of Spectacle Magnifiers

with the plano side toward the eye, the magnification will equal the Lensometer Power (which is the same as Equivalent Power in this special case) divided by 4. Such a lens, however, will have relatively poor optical performance, especially if the power is strong. The aberrations of astigmatism, curvature of field, distortion, and lateral chromatic aberration will combine to destroy image quality except at the very center of the field.

Let us see what happens if we combine two 40-diopter lenses.

EQUICONVEX (PAIRED)

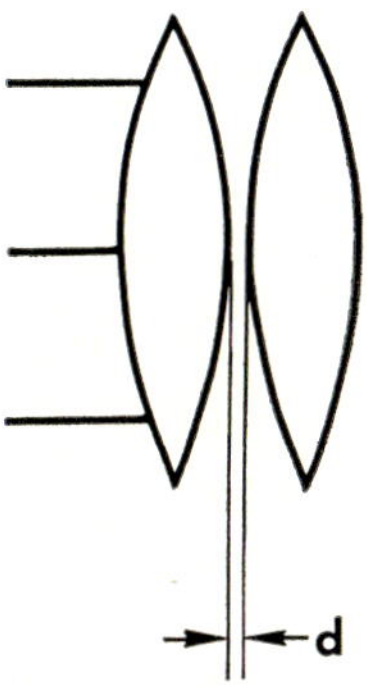

d	LENSOMETER POWER	EQUIVALENT POWER	MAGNIFICATION
0	128.16 Diop.	58.14 Diop.	14.5x
1	134.20	56.98	14.2
2	141.12	55.82	14.0
3	149.15	54.66	13.7
4	158.55	53.49	13.4
5	169.73	52.33	13.1

Figure VI-10. Two equiconvex +40 D lenses combined do not yield +80 D (17.0x) as expected, but only +58 D (14.5x). Power decreases as lenses are separated (d).

$$\text{WORKING DISTANCE} = \frac{1}{128.16} = .0078 \text{ METERS} = 7.8\text{MM} = .3 \text{ IN}$$

Figure VI-11. Lensometer Power is a measure of working distance. With the two 20-diopter equiconvex lenses, it is only 0.3 in.

Here we have two equiconvex, 40-diopter lenses, each of which, taken alone, would have a magnifying power of 8.5x. The combination, however, does not yield 17x as might be expected but only 14.5x (even less if the lenses are separated). But look at what has happened to the Lensometer Power. This is serious because Lensometer Power is a measure of working distance with parallel light on the ocular side of the system.

PLANOCONVEX (PAIRED)

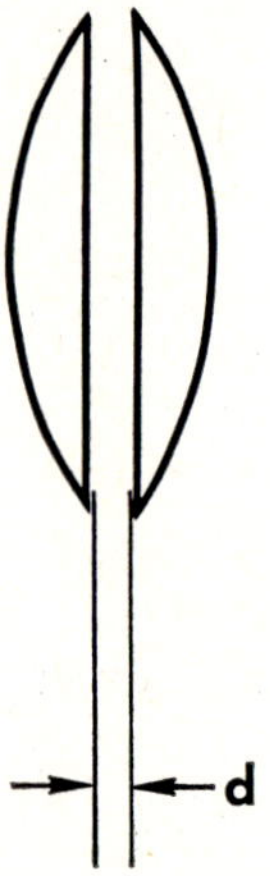

d	LENSOMETER POWER	EQUIVALENT POWER	MAGNIFICATION
0	89.11 Diop.	45.87 Diop.	11.5x
1	92.79	44.96	11.2x
2	96.95	44.04	11.0x

Figure VI-12. With the combined planoconvex +40 D lenses, the magnification is only 11.5x with a working distance of 0.4 in. Power decreases as the lenses are separated (d).

PLANOCONVEX, REVERSED (PAIRED)

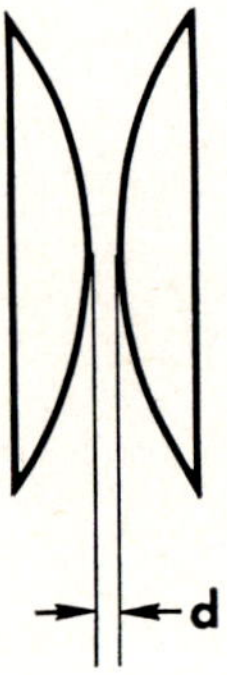

d	LENSOMETER POWER	EQUIVALENT POWER	MAGNIFICATION
0	222.75 Diop.	80.00 Diop.	20.0x
1	236.17	78.40	19.6x
2	251.98	76.80	19.2x

$$\text{WORKING DISTANCE} = \frac{1}{222.75} = .0045 \text{ METERS} = 4.5 \text{MM} = .18 \text{ IN}$$

Figure VI-13. Using two reversed planoconvex lenses of +40 D, the magnification is 20x, but the working distance is unfortunately only 0.18 in. Aberrations are well controlled with this system.

Let us look at what happens when we combine other lens configurations of the 40-diopter lenses. The situation here is similar. We have gained little in terms of magnification (11.5x for two in combination, as compared with 7.6x for a single lens) and have a working distance of only 11 mm (.4 inches).

Here we have doubled the magnification by combining two lenses. This is actually a pretty good magnifier except for one thing. Examine the working distance. The short working distance is especially unfortunate in this case, for otherwise the magnifier performs quite well indeed. Even the off-axis aberrations are fairly well under control.

So what is the answer? Is the situation hopeless? Certainly not. But as stated in the beginning, the designer's task is not simple. One approach in recent times has been to work with a single element lens, choose overall curvatures which yield suitable magnifications at useable working distances, and then optimize the aberrations through the use of aspheric curves. Although such curves are difficult to fabricate and inherently expensive, the use of plastic lens materials has made aspheric surfaces economically feasible for ophthalmic application. Further design sophistication, probably employing multiple aspheric surfaces, holds promise for future development.

· CHAPTER VII ·
Future Development of Optical Aids

Richard E. Feinbloom

Optical aids for the low vision patient have come a long way in the last five years. In the past, distance optical aids, telescopes, were only 2x in power, and only a few models were available: The Designs for Vision 2.2x Full-diameter Telescope; the Kollmorgen 2.2x Full-diameter Telescope, the Univis 2.0x Telescope and the Keeler 2.0x Telescope. Subsequently, Designs for Vision developed a 3.0x power and 4.0x power telescope and is now working on a new 6.0x power telescope made of glass.

Originally spectacle telescopes were mounted in the center of the carrier lens and decentered to the patient's distance P.D. In this position the patient's movements were greatly restricted. One can simulate this activity by looking through a pair of binoculars and trying to walk around. To overcome this problem of mobility, Designs for Vision produced its Bioptic 2.2x Model I Telescope. This rectangular telescope is designed to be positioned high in the spectacle lens so that the patient can look underneath and to the sides to get his bearings when walking around. When the patient has to spot some specific thing clearly, he simply tilts his head to look through the telescope. Placing the telescope in this configuration as high as possible in the spectacle lens permits the patient to make use of his peripheral vision.

Another major development in the past years which will help to guide us in the future was the introduction of aspheric and doublet lenses for reading. American Optical and Combined Optical Industries Limited produced a wide range of aspheric magnifying lenses for the low vision patient. The advantage of the aspheric lens over the spherical lens is better definition in the periphery of the field. The doublet lens system devised by Designs for Vision that has

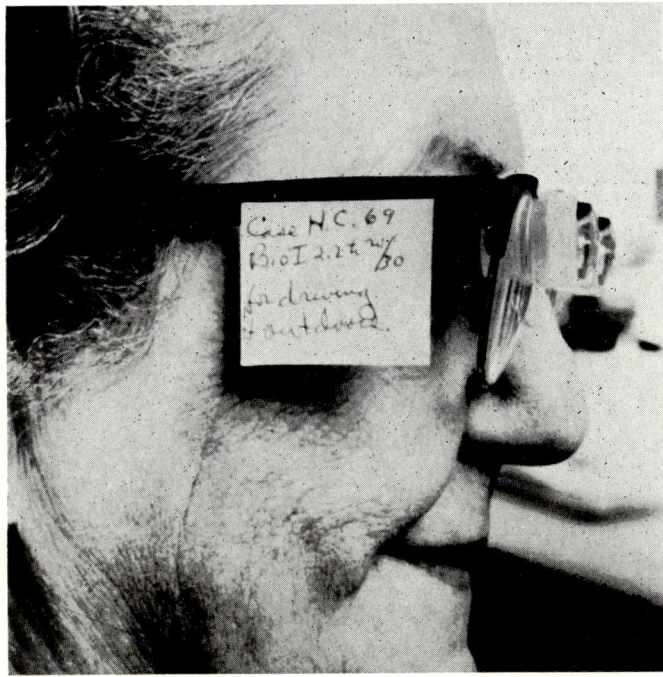

Figure VII-1. The Bioptic I 2.2x Telescope is positioned high in the carrier so that the patient has a full field when he is not looking through the telescopic unit.

an air space between two planoconvex spherical lenses increases the working distance and depth of focus with better aberration correction. These lenses are designed for near vision.

Recently, vision in the intermediate area, between distance and near, has been improved with telescopes fitted with low-power reading caps. This combination can give the same magnification as a near aid with a much greater working distance. The working distance of an afocal telescope fitted with a cap is the working distance of the lens in the cap.

Higher power, better resolution, a wider field, a longer working distance, these have been and continue to be the patient's needs and the designer's goals. Certainly one has heard the patient ask, Can't you make the field bigger? This is the simplest question, yet the hardest thing to do. If all one needs is a bigger field, just make the visual aid bigger. However, if we double the size of the system by using the same material, we have at least tripled its weight. This is why the field of view of present day optical systems is small. Optical aids of 2 power or more give a monocular field of 20° or less. If the field were to be doubled, the resulting weight of the system would be too much for the patient to wear in a frame.

The more compact a system, the lighter it becomes because less overall material is used. New types of raw glass with higher indices of refraction and special transmitting properties are becoming available to the system designer. These glasses will permit new systems with shorter overall axial lengths and better resolution. The material cost, however, can be considerably greater. For example, SK-16 glass which can be used for making eye lenses costs approximately ninety-six dollars per pound, as compared with BK-7 which costs approximately ten dollars per pound.

We are just beginning to use different forms of plastic for telescopic systems. Plastics already play an important part in near aids and spectacle lenses. Because of its lower index of refraction (1.47 to 1.50 compared to 1.53 to 2.0 for glass) and its shrinking proper-

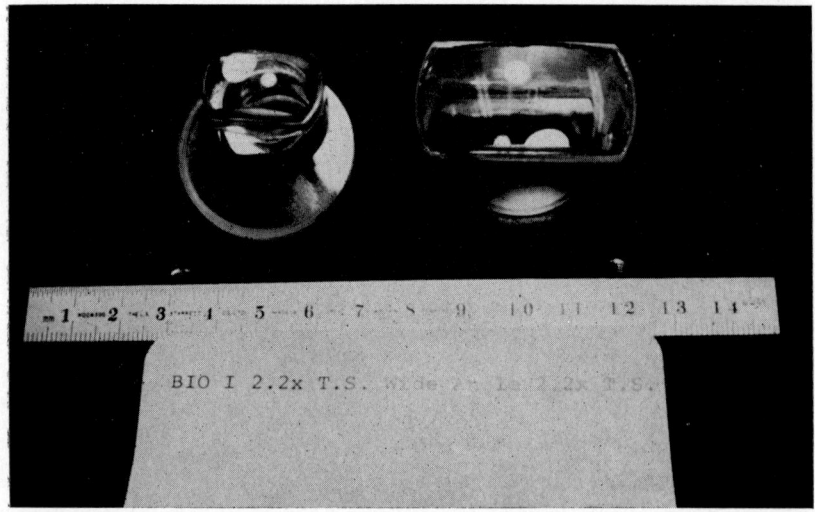

Figure VII-2. The 2.2x glass Bioptic I on the left has a field of 12°. The plastic objective 2.2x wide angle unit has a field of 17°. Patients more readily accept a larger field.

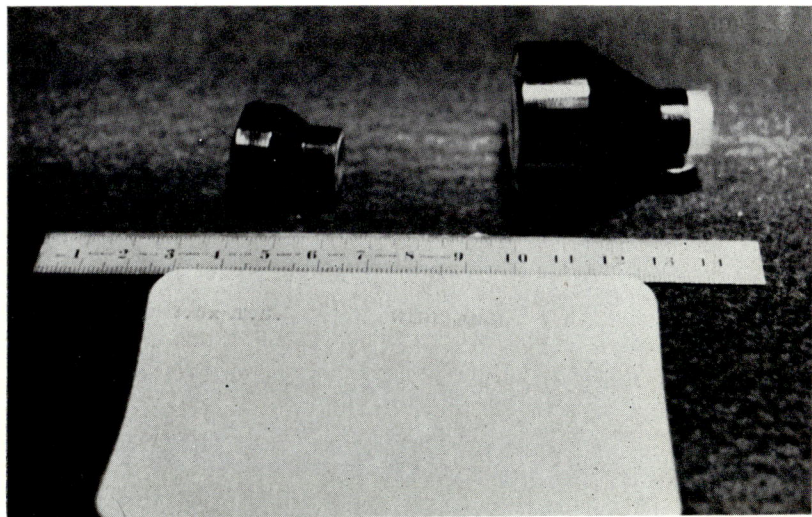

Figure VII-3. The 3x wide angle telescope on the right has an increased field of view of 11° compared with the older model on the left with a field of 8°. The wide angle lens is bulky.

ties, plastic was a poor choice of material for objective lenses. However, with some of the new glass available for the eye lens, plastic objectives can be combined in a system giving new, larger visual fields with good resolution.

The Designs for Vision 2.2x Wide Angle Telescope is an example. This plastic objective wide angle telescope gives a monocular field of 17° compared to the 12° field of the glass 2.2x telescope; yet the weight difference is insignificant, 21 gr compared to 19 gr. Although this new design is not the most cosmetically appealing, the patient accepts this aid readily because of the increased visual field. In fact, the success of this system spurred the development of the new 3.0x Wide Angle Telescope.

With the 3.0x Wide Angle Telescope we tried a new design concept of using two plastic meniscus lenses for the objective and a cemented doublet for the eye lens. This design increased the field of view of our standard 3-power telescope from 8° to 11°. In comparison, the weight went from 11 gr to 17 gr.

Stronger magnification also has its trade-offs. Many times the patient will choose an aid of weaker power because of the bigger field, longer depth of focus, and better resolution of the system due to more illumination. When one increases the magnification of an optical system, one decreases the area of the field. If the illumination remains constant in the field, less light is gathered through the optical system because one is viewing a smaller area. This loss in light affects the system by decreasing its resolution, thereby decreasing the visual acuity of the patient. The optical designer tries to compensate for this loss in light by designing larger light-gathering objective lenses. Yet he is handicapped because as he increases the diameter of the system, he increases the axial length and weight. The stronger the magnification, the greater the number of optical elements needed. This problem is a difficult one that the designer is constantly trying to overcome. This is why plastic offers the greatest possibilities in the future.

Every optical aid from the simple hand magnifier to the sophisticated closed-circuit television system has a focal point. At this point the system is at its sharpest focus. The distance from this point to the objective lens is the focal length. The depth of focus is the distance on either side of the focal point at which the object can still be clearly seen. The shorter focal length brought about by an increase in the magnification causes a decrease in the depth of focus of an optical system. Holding material within the narrow range at which the focus is clear can present quite a problem to the patient. Unless this is properly explained and accepted, the patient may never learn to use the optical aid properly.

Conventional high plus adds have shorter focal lengths but *greater depth of focus*. Technically the focal length of a +6.00 hand magnifier is 6.6 in. For a +20 hand magnifier the focal length is 2 in. The 10x microscopic lens has a focal length of 1 in. If the patient holds the object or reading material at the proper distance from the lens, this material will be in focus. If it is very hard for the elderly to hold their hands at the close fixed distance of a telescope, the use of a spectacle or hand held lenses which have a greater depth of focus is recommended. Telescopes with reading caps have greater focal lengths than conventional high plus near aids of the same magnification but have the disadvantage of having a restricted depth of focus. The +20 hand magnifier with a focal length of 2 in magnifies

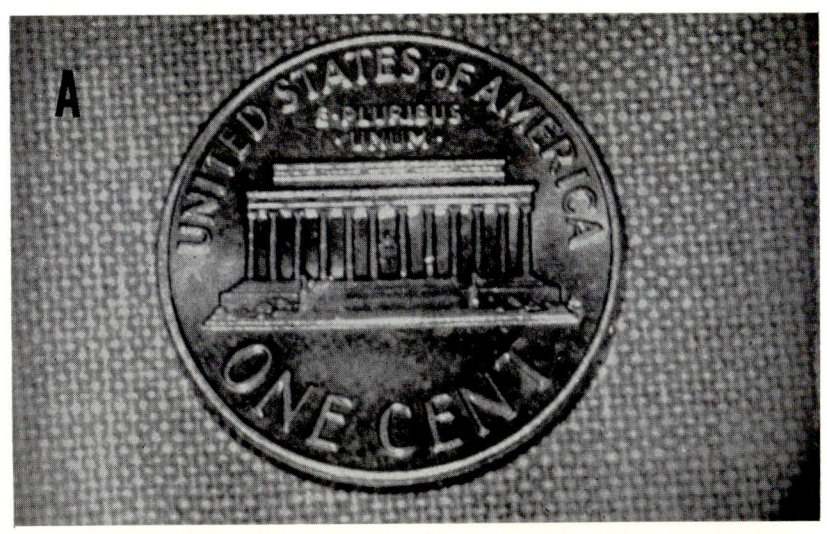

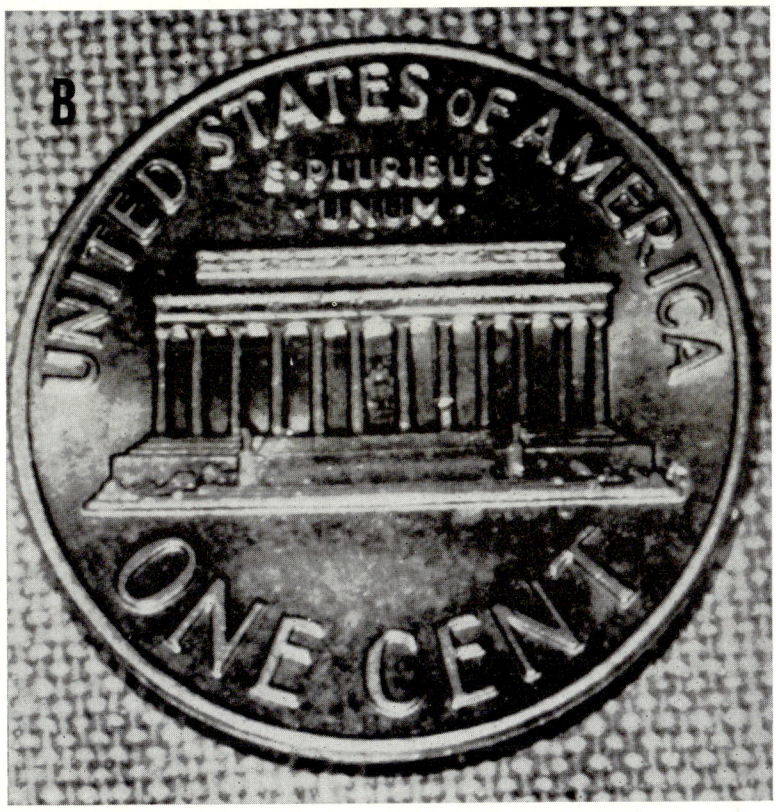

Figure VII-4 A & B. As magnification increases, field is decreased. To demonstrate this principle 4A views a penny with 2.2x magnification, 4B with 3x magnification.

Figure VII-4 C. A penny with 4x magnification.

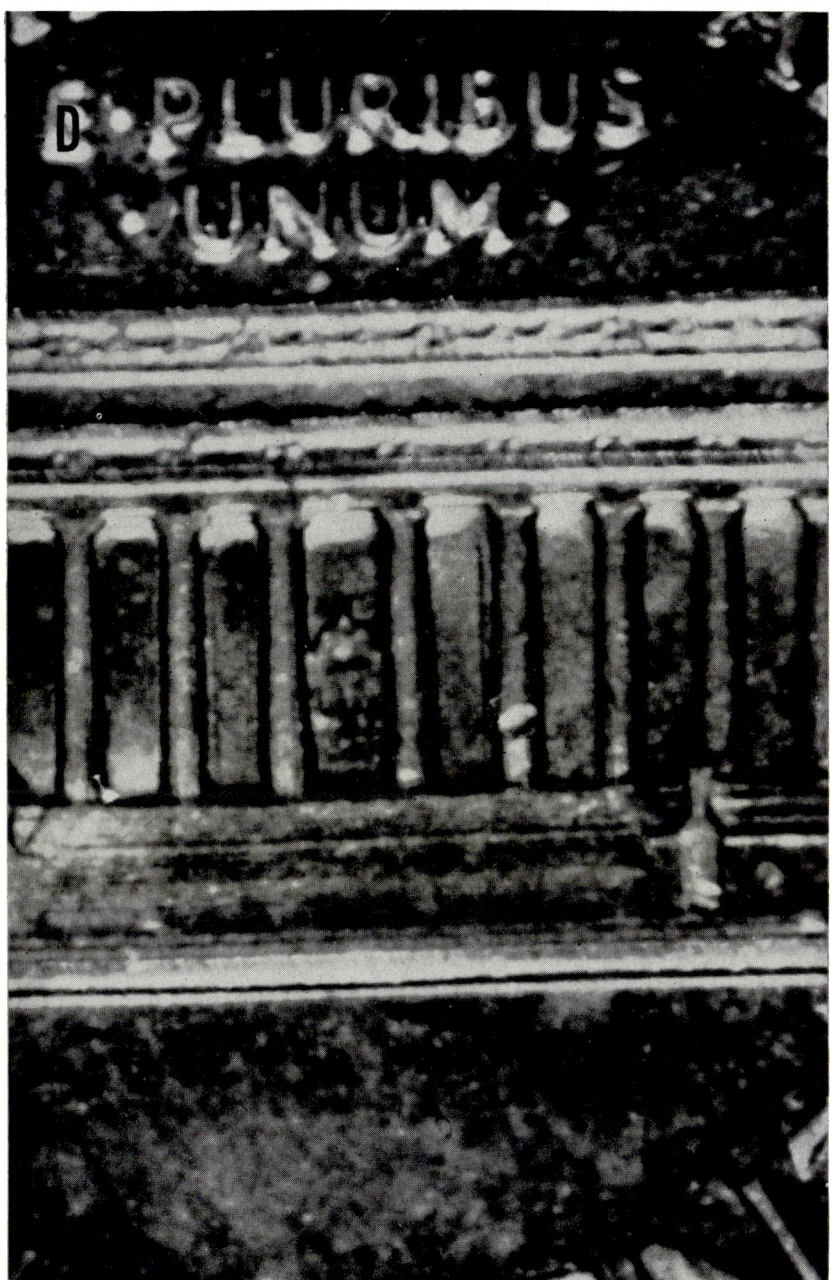

Figure VII-4 D. A penny with 6x magnification.

five times. The 4x telescope with a +5.00 diopter reading cap also magnifies five times but has a greater focal length of 8 in. In this case the advantage of the greater focal length to the patient has to be weighed against the higher unit cost and the decreased depth of focus as well as the smaller field.

But must this cost be greater? My answer as a manufacturer is no. As the field of low vision expands, more help will be given to a greater number of people. Greater volume should lower prices. Manufacturing techniques and new materials can result in lower overall costs. As an example, we designed for the New York Lighthouse a new series of high add bifocal lenses in 1-diopter steps from +5.00 to +12.00 diopters. These can be priced competitively with regular plastic bifocal spectacle lenses.

The systems we *design* today can exceed our ability to manufacture. We designed a plastic aspheric 6x Galilean telescope which, on paper, looked excellent. However, after contacting manufacturers of precision plastic lenses both in the United States and abroad, no one had the capability of making the lenses. In time, we hope that manufacturers will be able to meet such design objectives.

The designer and manufacturer are but one part of the low vision field. Seminars such as this one bring together people who are involved in the different facets of low vision and help all of us to have a better understanding of this field.

· SECTION THREE ·
Surgical and Medical Advances in Ophthalmology Related to the Low Vision Patient

· CHAPTER VIII ·

Latest Advances In Ophthalmic Surgery: Implications For the Low Vision Patient*

Norman B. Medow

Introduction

THE DAWN of recorded ophthalmic surgical history dates back to the ninth century B.C. when an Indian physician named Susruta removed a cataract from the visual axis of a low vision patient by a technique known as couching.[1]

Much surgical knowledge has been gained since that time, and advances such as the discovery of anesthesia by Morton in 1845,[2] antibiotics in 1936,[3] and cortisone in the 1940s[4] have allowed surgical results to be greatly improved.

When we speak about recent advances in ophthalmic surgery, one innovation stands out as being the guiding light for the development of our most recent techniques namely, the use of the operating microscope. It was not until the late 1950s that the operating microscope was proposed for use in ophthalmic surgery. The increased use of the microscope led to the development of fine surgical instruments and suture material to be used under the higher magnification of the operating microscope. This in turn opened the way for newer developments in every area of ophthalmic surgery.

In the broad field of ophthalmic surgery the following four areas are relevant to the low vision patient:

1. Keratoplasty.
2. Prosthokeratoplasty.

---

* The author wishes to thank the following people for their help in preparing this paper: Dr. Richard Troutman, Dr. Hernando Cardona, Dr. Nicholas Douvas, and Dr. Charles Kelman.

3. Cataract.
4. Vitrectomy.

Before planning ophthalmic surgery, a detailed history of the illness, medications used, reports from previous physicians, and a detailed examination is essential to establish an accurate diagnosis. There are two very important new tools in the diagnostic field with which the ophthalmic community should be familiar:

1. Ultrasonography.
2. Electroretinography.

When confronted with a patient whose cornea is opaque secondary to injury, infection, or disease one often cannot evaluate the other structures in the patient's eye. Is there a cataract present? Has the retina been damaged? Is there a foreign body within the eye? Is the vitreous clear, or has there been a vitreous hemorrhage?

Ultrasonography, a technique developed in 1957,[5,6] has afforded us a means of answering these questions. Basically, an ultrasonic wave is sent into the eye, and as it passes through the various portions of the inner aspects of the eye, it will return echoes of any diseased area that it traverses. These echoes are recorded on a display screen which may be photographed for use as a permanent record to document pathological changes in the interior of the eye.

Electroretinography[7] is another technique helpful in determining the level of function of the retina. When stimulated with light, an action potential is produced by the retina which, by using a corneal contact lens connected to an electrode, may be recorded on an oscilloscope. Diseases such as retinitis pigmentosa give typically absent or greatly subnormal electrical responses.

Keratoplasty

The first successful corneal transplant was performed by Von Hippel in 1888[8]. Few advances were made in corneal surgery until the 1930s, and although today's techniques vary from surgeon to surgeon, all have basic technical goals of obtaining a perfectly symmetrical donor button and suturing it exactly into place with fine suture material.

Still controversial and undergoing continual reevaluation and development are: (a) partial or through-and-through trephination;

(b) preoperative vitrectomy in aphakic bullous keratopathy; and (c) fresh vs preserved donor material and methods of suturing.

Most surgeons today are using one of the following methods of suture placement:

1. Multiple interrupted radially placed sutures of 8-0 silk, 10-0 monofilament nylon, or 13-0 (22µ) suture material.
2. A single continuous suture of 9-0 nylon, 10-0 nylon, or 13-0 suture material with four interrupted sutures of 8-0 or 9-0 at 3-6-9-12 o'clock.
3. Double continuous suture of 9-0, 10-0, or 13-0 suture material in an attempt to decrease the tortional and overriding tendencies of the graft.

It is generally agreed that the results of keratoplasty vary according to the pathological condition of the recipient's cornea.[9] Corneal diseases such as keratoconus, corneal scars secondary to trauma, and some of the corneal dystrophies have the best prognosis with a success rate of 90 percent. Aphakic bullous keratopathy, chemical and acid burns, as well as pathological conditions such as Stevens-Johnson syndrome bring the success rate down to 50 percent or less.

Complications in keratoplasty include graft rejection, glaucoma, cataract formation, and astigmatism.

The future of keratoplasty includes the development of an automated surgical trephine for obtaining even more precise corneal grafts; the development of suture material and closure methods; as well as continued research on methods of preserving corneas.

Prosthokeratoplasty

In the late 1950s Dr. Hernando Cardona[10] began the development of a keratoprosthesis for use in the opaque corneas of repeated graft failures and for diseases whose reactions to keratoplasty had always been notoriously poor. The keratoprosthesis he developed in the 1960s went through many more years of trial and modification until the present time at which there are two keratoprosthetic devices in use.[11,12,13]

One is for use in severely vascularized corneas and in eyes with loss of lacrimal function as well as conjunctival glandular function—examples of these are severe chemical burns and xerosis with its varied etiologies. This keratoprosthesis is a central optical cylinder with a surrounding perforated teflon plate. The power of the cylinder is determined by ultrasound,[14] and the surgical technique used is described elsewhere.[15]

The other keratoprosthesis is used in less severely vascularized corneal diseases such as aphakic bullous keratopathy. This prosthesis is called the nut-and-bolt type and consists of a mushroom-shaped bolt with a central optical cylinder and a cosmetic upper outer surface. The nut is perforated flexible teflon plate, and the surgical procedure used is described elsewhere.[16]

The results of both of these procedures are quite encouraging for patients who in former years were consigned to blindness. For many patients who presently have opaque corneas, a thorough reevaluation (including ultrasonography and electroretinography) may offer hope of regaining some residual vision. Complications include extrusion, (which has hopefully been brought to an acceptable minimum with the new prothesis) glaucoma, and retroprosthetic membranes.

Cataract

The history of cataract surgery is the history of ophthalmology itself. From the early days of couching to the developments of today, the cataract extraction has been the most often performed intraocular procedure, with approximately 400,000 cataract extractions done yearly.

In 1961 Dr. Krwawicz[17] of Poland developed the cryogenic (freezing) probe which formed a firm adhesion to the cataractous lens, thus enabling the intracapsular lens to be removed from the eye with a higher incidence of success than had been encountered with the various forceps used, especially in mature cataracts.

The standard cataract operation today is one in which a corneoscleral section of from 140° to 180° is made and the lens removed with either a cryoprobe or forceps. The incision is then tightly closed with a varying number and type of sutures.

In 1967 Dr. Charles Kelman[18] developed a technique which uses a small 2 mm corneoscleral incision. The lens material is removed by an ultrasonic probe equipped with irrigation and aspiration devices. The incision is closed with one suture, the patient is discharged from the hospital on the next day, and he is allowed to return to his usual activities almost immediately. This procedure is called phacoemulsification. To date, over seven thousand such procedures have been performed throughout the country. The procedure cannot be performed on all types of cataracts, and evaluation of each case is needed to determine if it can be done in this manner. What has been shown to date is the following:

1. Phacoemulsification is probably the procedure of choice in congenital and developmental cataracts in people under forty.
2. The older patients with mature or brunescent cataracts probably are not candidates, especially if they have any of the following:
    a. Shallow anterior chamber.
    b. Endothelial dystrophy.
    c. Subluxated lenses.
    d. Poorly dilated pupils.

The visual results in this procedure appear to be comparable to the standard types of cataract surgery.[19] One of the advantages of this type of surgery is the ability of the eye to tolerate a contact lens earlier than with the standard incision.

What appears to be very interesting is the following: although the loss of vitreous in the phacoemulsification procedure seems higher than in the standard cataract operation—3 to 5 percent for standard and 7 to 9 percent for phacoemulsification. The retinal detachment rate seems to be opposite (3 to 5% for standard cataract operations and less than 1% for phacoemulsification). It is felt that leaving the posterior capsule in place in the emulsification technique is perhaps protective.

In the standard intracapsular extractions, the rupture of the zonules in delivering the lens may produce significant trauma to the peripheral retina and thus set up the increased incidence of detachment.

Other variations in this procedure[20] are presently under development.

Vitrectomy

Prior to 1960, few surgeons would attempt a direct surgical approach to the vitreous.[21] In the late 1960s the cataract surgeons led the way to vitrectomy techniques when they began removing vitreous lost during cataract surgery. Techniques were developed to remove all of the vitreous from the anterior segment of the eye in hopes of decreasing the complication of vitreous wound entrapment, updrawn pupils and vitreous strands with traction on the retina,[22] and subsequent detachment.

In 1968 Dr. Kasner, et al.[23] removed vitreous from a primary vitreous disease, amyloidosis, and the era of the vitrectomy was entered.

In 1971 Dr. R. Machemer[24] developed an instrument known as the VISC, vitreous infusion suction cutter, which ushered in the era of the mechanical vitrectomy.

Since that time a number of instruments and techniques have been developed for surgical vitrectomy, [25,26,27] and Dr. Machemer has modified his.[28] The instruments are basically utilized in a similar manner in that an incision is made in the pars plana, the instrument is inserted into the vitreous, and under direct viewing either through the pupil or via a contact lens, the diseased vitreous is located, cut, and aspirated. The instruments differ in the type of cutting edge they have. Some are rotary, others are side and end cutting.

Indications for vitrectomy via these techniques vary but are generally used for vitreous hemorrhages either secondary to trauma, diabetes, or neovascular retinopathy of other etiologies, as well as primary vitreous disease.[29] The results are very encouraging for low vision patients who have an opaque vitreous and evidence of a retina which still is capable of functioning. (See ultrasonography and electroretinography).

Summary

A few of the most recent surgical techniques available for corneal, cataract, and vitreous surgery have been described. But what of the retina? To date, very little has been done in the field of direct attack on retinal pathology, photocoagulation being the only modality used for directly treating pathological conditions of the retina.

In Dr. Eleanor Faye's book, *The Low Vision Patient*,[30] Dr. Faye reviewed six thousand patients who were seen at the Low Vision Clinic during the years 1953 to 1963. In this group 50 percent of the patients had primary pathology of the retina. It is towards this group of people that our future research efforts should be directed.

REFERENCES

1. Stallard, H. B.: *Eye Surgery*. Baltimore, Williams and Wilkins, 1965, p. 519.
2. Atkinson, W. S.: *Anesthesia in Ophthalmology*. Springfield, Thomas, 1965, p. 3.
3. Goodman, L. S., and Gilman, A.: *The Pharmacological Basis of Therapeutics*. Macmillan, 1970, pp. 1154-1155.
4. Goodman, L. S., and Gilman, A.: *The Pharmacological Basis of Therapeutics*. Macmillan, 1970, pp. 1604-1605.
5. Goldberg, R. E., and Sarin, L. K.: *Ultrasonics in Ophthalmology*. Philadelphia, Saunders, 1967, pp. 10-11.
6. Goldberg, R. E., and Sarin, L. K.: *Ultrasonics in Ophthalmology*. Philadelphia, Saunders, 1967, pp. 45-75, 102-22.
7. Moses, R. A.: *Adler's Physiology of the Eye*. St. Louis, Mosby, 1970, pp. 498-28.
8. Stallard, H. B.: *Eye Surgery*. Baltimore, Williams and Wilkins, 1965, p. 402.
9. Fine, M., and Forster, R. K.: Donor age in penetrating keratoplasty. *Arch Ophthalmol.*, 85:42, 1971.
10. Cardona, H., Castroviejo, R., and DeVoe, A. G.: The Cardona keratoprosthesis: first clinical evaluation. *XIX Concilium Ophthalmologicum*, 2:1211, 1962.
11. Cardona, H., Castroviejo, R., and DeVoe, A. G.: Present status of prosthokeratoplasty. *Am J Ophthalmol.* 68(4): 613, 1969.
12. Cardona, H., Castroviejo, R., and DeVoe, A. G.: Advances in prosthokeratoplasty, In *Corneal Grafting*. London, Butterworth. Plenum Pub., 1972, p. 313.
13. Cardona, H.: Personal Communication, 1973 (to be published).
14. Coleman, D. L., Jack, R. L., and Cardona, H.: Ultrasonic evaluation of eyes with keratoprosthesis. *Am J Ophthalmol.*, 74:543, 1972.
15. Cardona. H.: Personal Communication (to be published), presented at the American Academy of Ophthalmology meeting, Dallas, Texas, 1973.
16. Cardona, H.: Personal Communication (to be published), presented at the American Academy of Ophthalmology meeting, Dallas, Texas, 1973.
17. Krwawicz, T.: Intracapsular extraction of intumescent cataract by application of low temperature. *Brit J Ophthalmol, 45*:279, 1961.
18. Kelman, C. D.: Phacoemulsification and aspiration: A new technique of cataract extraction. *Am J Ophthalmol, 64*:23, 1967.
19. Kelman, C. D.: Phacoemulsification and aspiration of senile cataracts:

A comparative study with intracapsular extraction. *Can J Ophthalmol,* 8:24, 1973.
20. Shock, J. P.: Phacofragmentation and irrigation of cataracts. *Am J Ophthalmol,* 74:187, 1972.
21. Shafer, D. M.: The treatment of retinal detachment by vitreous implant. *Trans Am Acad Ophthalmol Otolaryngol, 61*:194, 1952.
22. Kasner, D.: Vitrectomy: a new approach to the management of vitreous loss. *High Ophth, 11*:304, 1968.
23. Kasner, D., Miller, G. R., Taylor, W. H., Server, R. H., and Norton, E. W. D.: Surgical treatment of amyloidosis of the vitreous. *Trans Am Acad Ophthalmol Otolaryngol,* 74:410, 1968.
24. Machemer, R., Parel, J. M., and Buettner, H.: A new concept for vitreous surgery I: instrumentation. *Am J Ophthalmol, 73*:1, 1972.
25. Straatsma, B., et al.: Stereotaxic vitrectomy. *Clinical Trends, II (8)*: 1973.
26. Douvas, N.: *The Roto-Extractor.* Personal Communication.
27. O'Malley, C., and Heintz, R.: Vitrectomy via the pars plana: a new instrument system. *Trans Pac Coast Otoophthalmol Soc, 53*:121, 1972.
28. Machemer, R.: Subtotal vitrectomy through the pars plana. *Trans Amer Acad Ophthalmol Otolarygol,* 77:192, 1973.
29. Norton, E. W. D.: A new concept for vitreous surgery III indications and results. *Am J Ophthalmol,* 74:1034, 1972.
30. Faye, E.: *The Low Vision Patient.* New York, Grune and Stratton, 1970.

· CHAPTER IX ·

Laser Treatment and Low Vision Anatomical Considerations

Norman C. Charles

Introduction

THE MEDICAL therapy of retinal disease is now passing through an era of great excitement, innovation, and optimism. With the expansion of our therapeutic armamentarium, the treatment of macular disorders is proceeding on a widespread and enthusiastic basis. Such a time, however, is also a time of great danger. I refer not only to the known and as yet unknown hazards of powerful, energy-releasing instruments, but also to the hazards common to any era of technical innovation wherein enthusiasm overshadows rationality and sloppy, wishful thinking replaces the scientific method.

Therapeutic Considerations in Laser Treatment

Accordingly, there are certain key considerations which must constantly be borne in mind.

1. Certain disorders have an excellent prognosis for spontaneous resolution whether treated or not. Most cases of central serous retinopathy, for example, are self-limited and demonstrate spontaneous improvement in visual acuity.[1] If light coagulation is administered during the initial four months of a patient's first attack wherein spontaneous resolution is likely, the clinician may be falsely convinced that his therapy has favorably influenced the course of the disease.

2. Certain disorders have a poor prognosis whether treated or not. An obvious example is that of a dry macular gliotic scar. No amount of light coagulation may be expected to improve diminished visual acuity inherent in such an irrevocable anatomic situation.

3. A variety of therapeutic modalities is available. Currently the most popular light coagulation devices are the xenon arc photocoagulator, the argon laser, and the ruby laser. Others, such as the krypton laser, are under laboratory evaluation. The choice of instrument should be based on such considerations as the experience and skill of the operator or the appropriate properties of the emitted beam in relation to the specific retinal derangement, rather than the newness or glamour of the instrument.

4. Whatever instrument is chosen, both physician and patient should understand that its usage to date is experimental in nature and that attendant risks are always present. Certain complications of light coagulation, chorioretinal hemorrhage or inadvertent coagulation of the fovea, are well known. Other complications may have yet to be defined.

The light coagulator is a double-edged sword. Its primary effect is the production of chorioretinal scarring for protective or therapeutic reasons. Yet chorioretinal scarring, in its locus of application, must necessarily destroy the visual pathway and the local capacity for transmission of the visual impulse. If extensive enough, a clinical scotoma may result.

Furthermore, it is conceivable that the delivery of high levels of energy to the retina may be discovered in the future to have deleterious effects, not only upon the disorder which has undergone treatment but even upon normal retina.

5. Further complicating the treatment of such diseases as senile disciform macular degeneration or diabetic retinopathy is the fact that the natural courses of such diseases are incompletely understood. While this fact does not obviate the need for treatment of the visually impaired patient, it does generate confusion in evaluating the optimal role of the light coagulator in therapy.

6. Even additional confusion stems from the observation that certain kinds of therapy are effective in producing a desired result although the biologic mechanism of therapeutic effectiveness remains obscure.

Principles and Treatment of Macular Derangements

Taking a rational approach to the fundamentals, I would now

like to demonstrate some of the anatomical principles involved in diagnosis and treatment of macular diseases. Obviously a comprehensive survey of this subject is impossible in this brief review, and I will limit my remarks only to certain derangements involving the macula and fovea, the area of the greatest visual acuity.

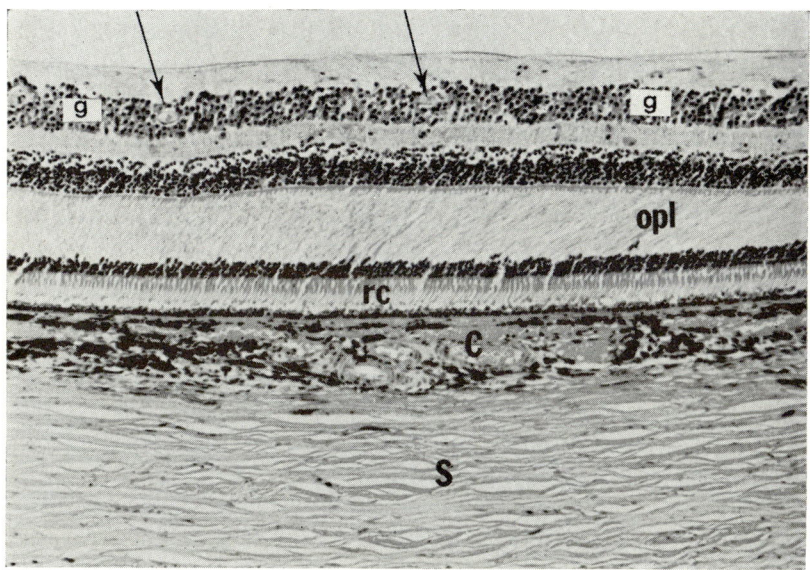

Figure IX-1. Normal human parafoveal macular area with thickened ganglion cell layer (g) and oblique arrangement of outer plexiform layer (opl). Both inner retinal vessels (arrows) and choroidal circulation (C) are present outside the fovea. Rod and cone layer (rc) contains increasing ratio of cones to rods near the fovea. Sclera (S). (Hematoxylin-eosin, x25).

The clinical macula is an apparently avascular area temporal to the disc. Centrally the foveal reflex is seen and is caused by the convergence of light rays by the inner concave foveal surface, a tiny concave mirror. Histologically the macula shows increase in ganglion cell layer from the usual one layer to 5-7 layers in thickness. Clinically the ganglion cell layer is transparent and invisible unless opacification occurs, as in such relatively rare pathologic states as central retinal artery occlusion, Tay Sachs disease, or Niemann-Pick disease. The normal macular area contains the complete number of retinal layers and is nourished by both inner retinal and choroidal circulation, although the fovea or point of greatest acuity shows absence of inner retinal layers and inner circulation. The outer plexiform layer of the macula shows a centrifugal or funnel-shaped arrangement of its fibers, so that laser destruction of retinal pigment epithelium at any point might produce a clinical scotoma slightly peripheral to the burn.

The abnormalities currently being treated are characterized by the passive accumulation of fluid in or near the foveo-macular area. If *in* the macula, one hopes for resorption of fluid; if *near* the macula, one hopes to protect the macula from involvement by laying down a barrier of chorioretinal scarring between the locus of fluid and the macula.

Three Groups of Macular Disorders—Treatment Objectives

Gass[1] has divided patients with loss of macular function secondary to retinal vascular disease into three groups. The first group shows accumulation of subretinal and intraretinal exudates in the macula secondary to *peripheral segmental* abnormal capillary permeability. An example of such a disorder would be Von Hippel's disease. Treatment, that is, the production of destructive scarring, is limited to a segment of retinal periphery, following which the macular fluid hopefully resorbs. If the treated segment is isolated or remote from the macula, the danger of producing a disabling scotoma is minimized.

A second group shows accumulation of exudate in the macular area secondary to *diffuse* retinal capillary abnormalities. Diabetes exemplifies such a condition. Here one may have to treat extensive areas of the fundus in the hope that macular fluid will resorb. Sometimes it does and sometimes it does not. Unfortunately it is difficult to predict success or failure *or* to explain the mechanism of the result obtained. Now, there is one rather disturbing thought in this situation; namely, if the production of extensive chorioretinal scarring has failed to bring about restoration of vision by resorption of macular fluid, then it may have also precluded the restoration of visual acuity with low vision optical aids by destroying viable paramacular and peripheral retinal areas.

The principle of magnification in low vision therapy involves projection of an enlarged image onto a retinal area whose center is

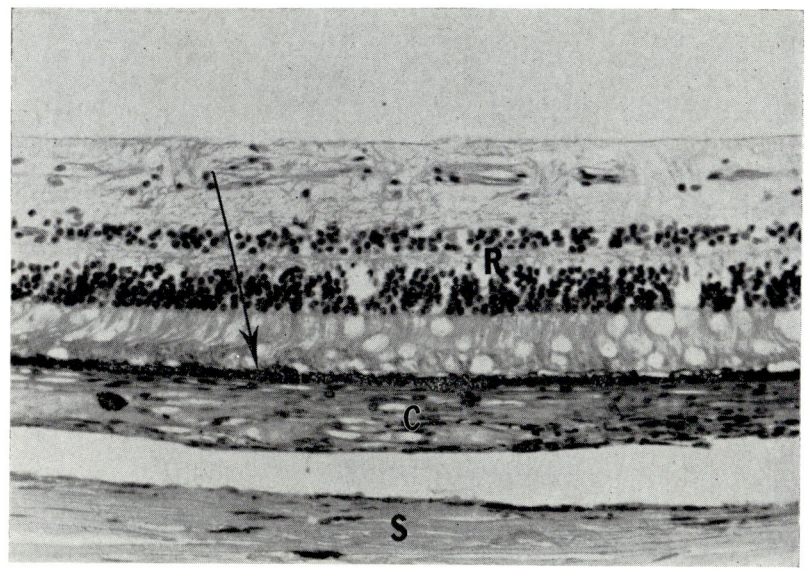

Figure IX-2A. Untreated area of peripheral human retina (R) in a diabetic, with intact retinal pigment epithelium (arrow). Sclera (S). Choroid (C). (PAS, x64).

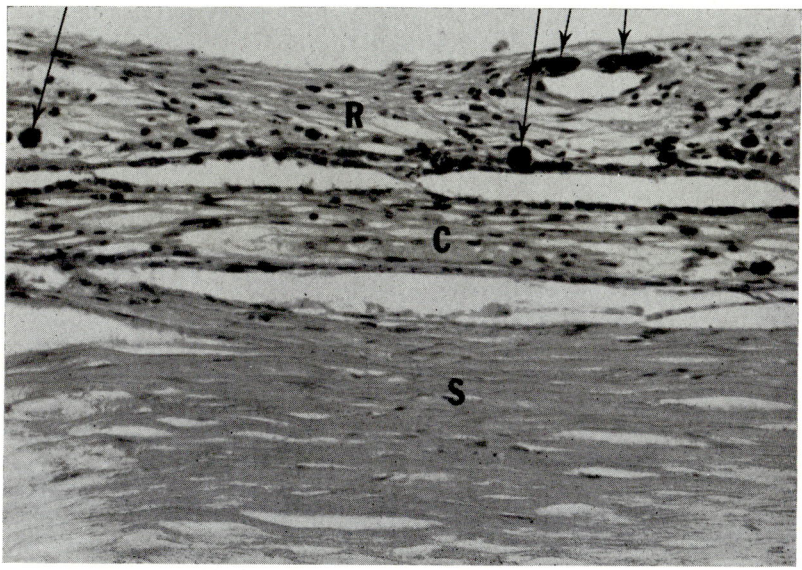

Figure IX-2B. Peripheral human retina in the same eye showing area treated with xenon photocoagulator. Marked destruction of retinal architecture (R) with intraretinal migration and proliferation of retinal pigment epithelium (arrows). Choroid (C). Sclera (S). (PAS, x64). (Case no. E 187-70, Bascom Palmer Eye Institute, courtesy of Dr. Henry Ring.)

the macula but whose radius extends well beyond the macula into more peripheral normal retina. It is conceivable that intense photocoagulation, if sufficiently destructive in area, may decrease the success of the low vision refraction.

The third group of disorders shows macular accumulation of exudate which is secondary to *local* vascular abnormalities immediately adjacent to the macular area, as in senile exudative maculopathy. One goal may be the photocoagulation and sealing of a leak which is demonstrable by fluorescein angiography. If the leak is not too close to the fovea and the sealing is done carefully with a small, not-too-intense beam, then the danger of inadvertently burning the fovea is minimal. If the leak is near the fovea or excessive photocoagulation is needed to seal it, one may be left with visual acuity worse than before treatment.

Another therapeutic goal might be barrier formation by a row of chorioretinal scars. Here we might expect little loss of visual field, but the possibility of disrupting the papillomacular bundle arises. It is generally agreed that intense photocoagulation of the papillomacular bundle should be avoided, as one can produce a centrocecal scotoma. It has been recently shown, however, that mild to moderate xenon and ruby laser coagulation of the papillomacular bundle in rhesus monkeys affects only the retinal pigment epithelium and outer retina and spares the nerve fiber layer.[2,3] Blair and Gass[4] also studied one human subject whose moderate photocoagulation in the papillomacular bundle was produced by the ruby and xenon photocoagulators. Visual fields were done showing no central or centrocecal scotoma. After exenteration for orbital tumor, histologic exam revealed destruction limited to the choroid and outer retina only.

Another goal in exudative senile retinopathy might be the treatment around the lesion in horseshoe pattern presumably to prevent spread of the exudate. The open part of the horseshoe faces the papillomacular bundle. Again, one wonders what benefits derive from such an alteration of mechanical forces. Perhaps the horseshoe barrier actually forces fluid *towards* the papillomacular bundle. Perhaps a horseshoe, especially a large one, reduces the area of viable paramacular retina needed for successful low vision refraction.

Treatment Based on Prognosis

Perhaps we also need to know when not to treat as based on prognosis. Clinical reports show that the best prognosis is associated with pure serous detachment of the neuroepithelium. The prognosis is much worse, on the other hand, with hemorrhagic detachment of retinal pigment epithelium, especially if subpigment epithelial neovascular membranes are present. Schatz[5] notes that, "If a patient has had a hemorrhagic detachment of the pigment epithelium and less than 6/200 visual acuity before treatment, he has virtually no chance for recovery of useful central visual acuity." In such a case, then, the patient may be worse after the treatment with the photocoagulator than before. Schatz also notes that the goal of obliterating subpigment epithelial neovascularization appears to be frustrating, as obliteration in one area may leave one with proliferation in other areas.

Summary

In summary, it appears obvious that both open-mindedness and greater experience in therapy of retinal diseases are necessary so that more precise criteria for treatment may be established. One hopes for more controlled objective studies in the future, and one might consider, as an example, the following proposed study of the effect of treatment on the low vision examination:

1. The selection of patients with a bilateral macular disorder.
2. The performance, prior to treatment, of visual fields, and the recording of bilateral near vision acuity, using a magnifying aid whose power is determined by the Kestenbaum method.
3. Light coagulation treatment of one eye only, when a horseshoe pattern or more extensive coagulation is planned.
4. Repetition of visual fields and the low vision refraction at suitable intervals following treatment.

Clearly such a study would involve much time and painstaking effort. Yet these are the dues which one pays for scientific progress.

REFERENCES

1. Gass, J. D. M.: Photocoagulation of macular lesions. *Trans Am Acad Ophthalmol Otolaryngol*, 75:580-08, 1971.

2. Townes, D. E., and Watzke, R. C.: Xenon photocoagulation of the papillomacular bundle. *Arch Ophthalmol, 87*:79-83, 1972.
3. Watzke, R. C., and Moore, R. T.: Ruby laser photocoagulation of the papillomacular bundle. *Arch Ophthalmol, 87*:684-87, 1972.
4. Blair, C. J., and Gass, J. D. M.: Photocoagulation of the macula and papillomacular bundle in the human. *Arch Ophthalmol, 88*:167-71, 1972.
5. Schatz, H., and Patz, A.: Exudative senile maculopathy. *Arch Ophthalmol, 90*:183-02, 1973.

· CHAPTER X ·
Argon Laser Coagulation (ALC)

Lawrence Yannuzzi

Introduction

OVER THE past few years Argon laser coagulation (ALC) has become an increasingly prominent modality in therapy of diseases of the macula and a variety of other vascular conditions involving the posterior segment of the eye. The unique properties of current laser instruments provide ophthalmologists with a monochromatic, coherent, and intense microbeam combined with a well-illuminated stereoscopic delivery system. Ophthalmologists now have the capability of producing a biological thermal response at the level of the retinal pigment epithelium or retinal vasculature that can be programed and reasonably well predicted. Unfortunately, notwithstanding this great technological innovation, the technique of Argon laser coagulation has a number of limitations as well as certain potential complications.

In selection of patients for treatment of a disease by a particular modality, clinicians usually call upon their understanding of a natural course of a disease and then compare this course to treated cases from well-documented, controlled, statistical studies with good experimental design. Unfortunately in ophthalmology the natural course of all these diseases is poorly understood at best. In addition, there is no current study involving any particular macular disease amenable to ALC that involves a large number of cases examined over a sufficient period of time that adequately compares *treated* with *nontreated* cases. In selection of patients for treatment, we are faced with a double-barrelled problem: a poor understanding of the natural course of the disease *and* a lack of clinical experience documenting the benefits of ALC.

This paper will review those diseases of the eye which are amenable to ALC, stressing the role of fluorescein angiography as a means for patient selection and as a guide to ultimate treatment. Those diseases in which Argon laser coagulation offers no therapeutic improvement will also be considered.

Evaluation of Patient

A complete systemic and ocular evaluation must be carried out in all candidates for ALC. Regulation of all metabolic disturbances, particularly the blood pressure, are of utmost importance. The visual acuity for near and distance, the central field exam, a good clinical exam with slit lamp biomicroscopy, the Goldmann lens, and the indirect ophthalmoscope are of equal importance as diagnostic procedures. Finally a thorough and recent pretreatment, stereo, rapid-sequential fluorescein angiogram is essential. Exudative vs nonexudative areas can be documented, and particular regions of neovascularization can be defined. It is the fluorescein angiogram that will ultimately determine the method and site of Argon laser coagulation.

Diseases Amenable to Light Coagulation

There are actually five major categories of diseases amenable to photocoagulation:
1. Retinal tears and separations.
2. Glaucoma.
3. Inflammations.
4. Pigment epithelial-Bruch's membrane-choroidal disease.
5. Retinal vascular diseases.

The principles of coagulation in tears and separations of the retina have been well established for a number of years. Glaucoma laser surgery on the other hand is still experimental. Except for presumed ocular histoplasmosis and rare ocular parasites, inflammations are seldom treated. The remaining two major categories, retinal vascular disease and pigment epithelial disease, will be discussed with particular reference to the macula.

Retinal Vascular

VENOUS OCCLUSIVE DISEASE. The first category under retinal

vascular diseases is *venous occlusive disease*. The technique of laser coagulation will vary depending on the site of the occlusion, the duration of occlusion, and the presence of secondary complications. Retinal branch vein occlusion in our experience usually responds dramatically to no treatment at all with ultimately good vision returning six to nine months after the event. Favorable factors associated with branch vein occlusions include early absorption of retinal blood, minimal intraretinal edema, adequate arteriolar perfusion, and thromboses which are distal to the immediate optic nerve area. Less favorable factors include alterations in the macular perfusion, macular preretinal membrane formation, persistent macular edema with cyst and hole formation, retinal and vitreous neovascularization, vitreous hemorrhage, sudden drop in the acuity following a transient improvement, and concomitant arteriolar insufficiency, particularly in elderly hypertensive patients. Argon laser coagulation should be considered only when these unfavorable factors begin to predominate. Then fluorescein angiogram is relied on for determination of the extent of the macular edema, the location of the neovascularization, the degree of capillary perfusion, and evidence of other occlusive phenomena. When there is inadequate capillary perfusion, cyst and hole formation of the macula, or preretinal membrane formation ALC serves no useful purpose. Persistent macular edema can be treated well with ALC under fluorescein angiographic guidance when the central vision is deteriorating after a period of improvement. Neovascularization adjacent to the disc may be approached utilizing a modified retinal ablation technique involving the entire segment of the retina at the site of the occlusion.

RETINAL PROLIFERATIVE DISEASE. Retinal proliferative disease may be classified as diabetic or nondiabetic. In the case of diabetic retinal problems, there are essentially three presentations to the clinical ophthalmologist. First, a diabetic may appear with background diabetic retinopathy with no evidence of proliferative or major occlusive disease. These nonproliferative cases when extensive may be treated with panretinal ablation utilizing 1000 to 1500 photocoagulation applications outside the major arcades to the equator of the eye. In cases of proliferative diabetic retinopathy, panablation is carried out as a primary technique to be followed in a period of two to four months with *selective* treatment of proliferating vascular fronds following fluorescein studies to demonstrate feeder vessels. The final category of diabetic disease is that of pure macular edema. In rare cases, diabetics present with minimal background retinopathy and pure macular cystoid edema. The fluorescein angiogram outlines the area of edema, and this area in turn is treated with direct coagulation. The prognosis for ultimate visual improvement is poor and is contingent on adequate macular capillary perfusion in the treated area.

VASCULAR PROLIFERATIVE NONDIABETIC DISEASE. Vascular proliferative nondiabetic diseases include microaneurysms, sickle cell hemoglobin SC disease, Eales's disease, and angiomatosis of the retina. After demonstration of the abnormal vascular proliferation with the fluorescein angiogram, direct coagulation can be carried out. It has been noted on a number of occasions that peripheral proliferative vascular changes associated with macular edema can be treated with ultimate absorption of the secondary exudative change that occurs at the site of the macula.

Extensive glial and fibrovascular proliferation of vessels from the surface of the disc, particularly in the region of the macula or into the vitreous associated with shallow detachments of the base of the vitreous, are all *contraindications* to treatment with Argon laser coagulation. There is a strong tendency towards hemorrhage into the vitreous when these conditions are treated. Well-entrenched neovascularization on the surface of the retina, particularly when associated with shallow detachments of posterior base of the vitreous, also set the stage for massive vitreous retraction and hemorrhage when coagulated.

Retinal Pigment Epithelial-Bruch's Membrane-Choroidal Disease

This category may be approached in terms of three major headings: (a) idiopathic central serous choroidopathy, (b) pure pigment epithelial detachments, and (c) involutional macular degeneration with serous or hemorrhagic detachment of the pigment epithelium and sensory retina (with or without subretinal neovascularization).

Central serous choroidopathy is a disease of particular interest. The author has accumulated 111 primary cases which have *not* been treated with Argon laser coagulation in an attempt to determine the natural course of this disease. Although the author, as well as other observers, has seen that spontaneous remission is generally the rule in the primary case, two observations have been made which appear to be significant. First, this is not a benign disease. A number of people have persistent subjective as well as objective findings following absorption of the fluid. Patients still complain of metamorphopsia after the fluid is absorbed, and there is often evidence of retinal pigment epithelial atrophy and pigmentary disturbance following complete disappearance of the fluid. The acuity disturbances as well as metamorphopsia and scotomas on Amsler Grid testing are also evident. The role of Argon laser coagulation is still not established. There is no question that ALC at the proper site of the focal abnormalities as demonstrated by fluorescein angiography does result in rapid elimination of the subneurosensory fluid when compared to time alone. The ultimate visual acuity and state of the eye with and without Argon laser coagulation treatment are still not clearly understood. Of principal importance in coagulation is the fact that only a light thermal reaction is required to treat these leaking areas. Accidental foveal burns or a scotoma from heavy coagulation are very rare complications in this disease.

Pure retinal pigment epithelial detachments can be documented on fluorescein angiographic examination. These must be differentiated from combined epithelial and sensory detachments by the angiogram, because photocoagulation is not needed in these epithelial detachments. They may persist for long periods without noticeable affect on the central vision.

Involutional macular degeneration is the prime category of diseases to be considered in this overall group. At the Manhattan Eye, Ear and Throat Hospital, this category has been subclassified as follows:

1. Nonexudative.
2. Exudative.
   a. Serous.
   b. Hemorrhagic detachment of the retinal pigment epithelium.
   c. Subretinal neovascularization (foveal or nonfoveal).

If the degenerative process is nonexudative in nature, no coagulation is necessary. This is determined by the fluorescein angiogram which shows no alteration in the permeability of the chorioretinal pigment epithelial barrier. This type of *dry* maculopathy is not aided by coagulation therapy. However, if the disease is exudative, it will have one or more of the following changes: serous detachment of retinal pigment epithelium, serous detachment of the sensory retina, hemorrhagic detachment of the retinal pigment epithelium, cystoid edema of detached sensory retina, and, finally, subretinal neovascularization. In the author's experience, any case with evidence of subretinal neovascularization anywhere in the macular region is seldom aided by light coagulation. When subretinal neovascularization can be demonstrated by fluorescein angiography, ALC will most likely serve no useful purpose, and, if given insufficiently may even serve to promote accelerated growth of the neovascularized complex and reduce acuity earlier than if the lesion were left untreated. The extent of the subretinal neovascularization is probably much greater than appreciated even with fluorescein angiography. If there is hemorrhagic detachment of the pigment epithelium, this can conceal a neovascularized membrane and absorb the Argon laser light excessively, and this would have secondary effects on the overlying nerve fiber layer in the sensory retina. The prognosis in an eye like this is extremely poor, and light coagulation should be avoided. In epithelial detachments which are pure serous but the turbidity or proteinaceous content of subpigment epithelial fluid is high, extreme coagulation is needed as in the hemorrhagic detachment; and this type of case is also doomed to failure. Only a fresh, pure epithelial detachment which has clear subpigment epithelial fluid and no evidence of subretinal neovascularization is likely to benefit from photocoagulation with Argon laser light. In these cases the epithelial detachment can disappear, improving at least the distant acuity. Massive coagulation of this region may sacrifice the near vision at the same time it improves the distance vision. The response to spectacle magnification in an eye in which extensive macular coagulation has been carried out is extremely variable. A study being conducted by Dr. Faye and the author will hopefully clarify some of the variables associated with this disparity between distance and near vision in this treatment.

Ocular Inflammations

Ocular histoplasmosis has proved to be of great importance in Argon laser coagulation. Provided that accurate and complete identification of subretinal areas of fibrovascular proliferation can be determined with a fluorescein angiogram, intense coagulation with Argon laser light can be carried out successfully with elimination of exudative detachments, exudative and hemorrhagic detachments, and restoration of central vision. This is truly an area where ALC offers hope as a primary treatment in the management of this disease.

Summary

The role of the laser in macular disease has been briefly reviewed. There are difficulties in patient selection due to limitations in knowledge of the natural course of macular diseases. Studies to determine the true value of laser coagulation in this area are needed. In the future, studies on the natural course of these diseases as well as controlled studies on treatment vs nontreatment are necessary to indicate what the laser can do and what its therapeutic potential may be.

· SECTION FOUR ·

Field Defects and Optical Management

CHAPTER XI

Neuro-Ophthalmological Defects in the Partially Sighted Patient

Thomas R. Kuhns

Disturbances in the visual sensory system are manifested by loss of visual acuity and color discrimination or defects in the visual field. The physician managing a partially sighted patient must not only have an understanding of the ocular pathology but also the primary visual sensory defect that is incapacitating the patient.

Four Groups of Visual Defects

Patients with defects in the visual sensory system may be generally classified into four groups. These groups present their special problems and methods of management.

The First Group: Loss of Central Visual Acuity. The patients have central scotomas and complain of difficulty in reading and fixing on small objects.

The macular degenerations are the most common retinal etiology. The neurological causes may be optic neuritis or nutritional amblyopia. Only a small area of retina has to be damaged to markedly reduce visual acuity. Vision is already reduced to 20/100, 10° from the center of the fovea, a radius of only 3.0 mm.

The solution to the reading problem for these patients is to magnify the image around their central scotoma. This is accomplished by using high plus magnifiers or spectacles. The patient has often adopted a head turn to use his peripheral vision.

The Second Group: Loss of Peripheral Field. These patients complain of difficulty finding the object of regard in their limited field. This small field adversely affects reading continuity as well as orientation and mobility. The most common causes of these defects are glaucoma and pigmentary degeneration of the retina.

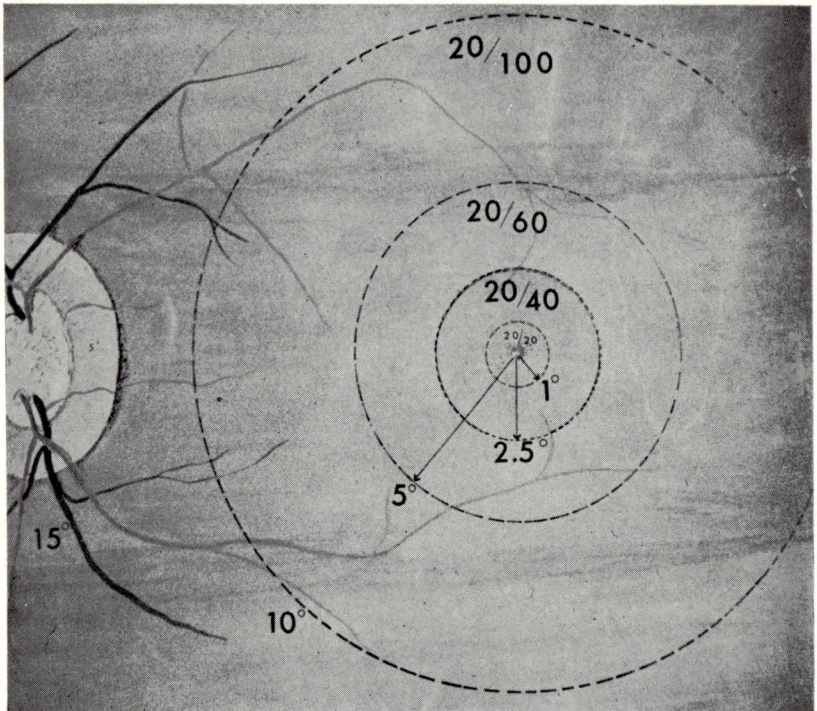

Figure XI-1. A map of the macular area demonstrates the visual acuity in the surrounding zones. The foveolar radius is 0.5°. The rod-free area radius is 1°. The fovea is 2.5°. The macular radius is 5°. At a radius of 10° from the foveola, vision falls to 20/100.

The problem for these patients is that the field of vision is too small to appreciate a magnified image. A hand magnifier held away from the eye so the image is not lost in the constricted field is helpful.

THE THIRD GROUP: FIELD DEFECTS OF NEUROLOGICAL DISEASE. The problems these patients experience are in recognizing and adjusting to their field loss. The altitudinal hemianopias occur most commonly with ischemic optic neuropathies. Homonymous hemianopias occur with retrochiasmal neoplastic and vascular disease. These patients are usually hospitalized as diagnostic problems and often are critically ill.

Inferior altitudinal defects are more common and more incapacitating to reading and mobility than superior altitudinal hemianopias.

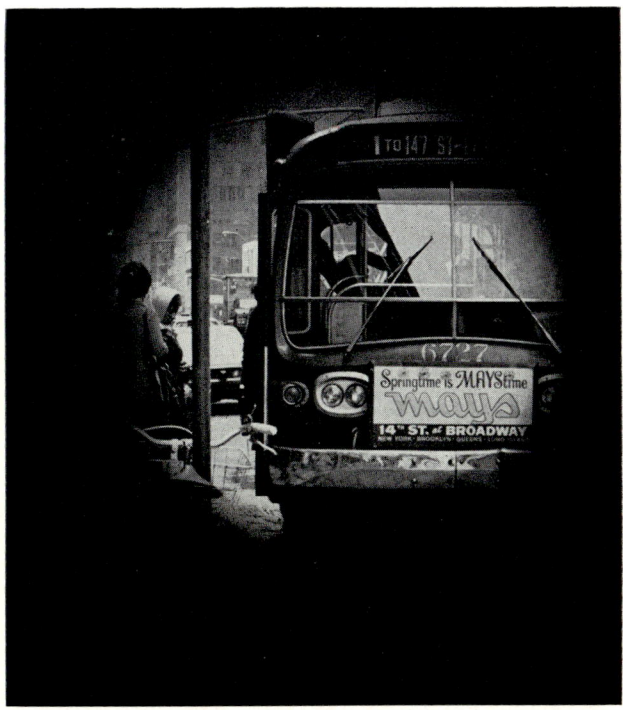

Figure XI-2. Reduced peripheral field interferes with mobility, orientation, and the appreciation of magnified objects.

Right homonymous hemianopias interfere with reading more than left field defects. Driving safety is limited by all hemianopias especially bitemporal hemianopias of chiasmal lesions.

These patients may be instructed to adapt to their field loss by head turns and in some cases prism devices and special mirrors mounted on spectacles or held by hand to reflect the area of the missing field. This adaptive teaching is often neglected during the rehabilitation period when survival is the primary concern.

THE FOURTH GROUP: DIFFUSE LOSS OF VISION. This is the most frustrating type of visual loss for the patient to adjust to and the physician to manage. This loss of vision is characterized by sudden exacerbations and slow remissions.

The common causes are hemorrhagic diabetic retinopathy, vitreous hemorrhages, and uveitis. Temporary magnifying devices may be

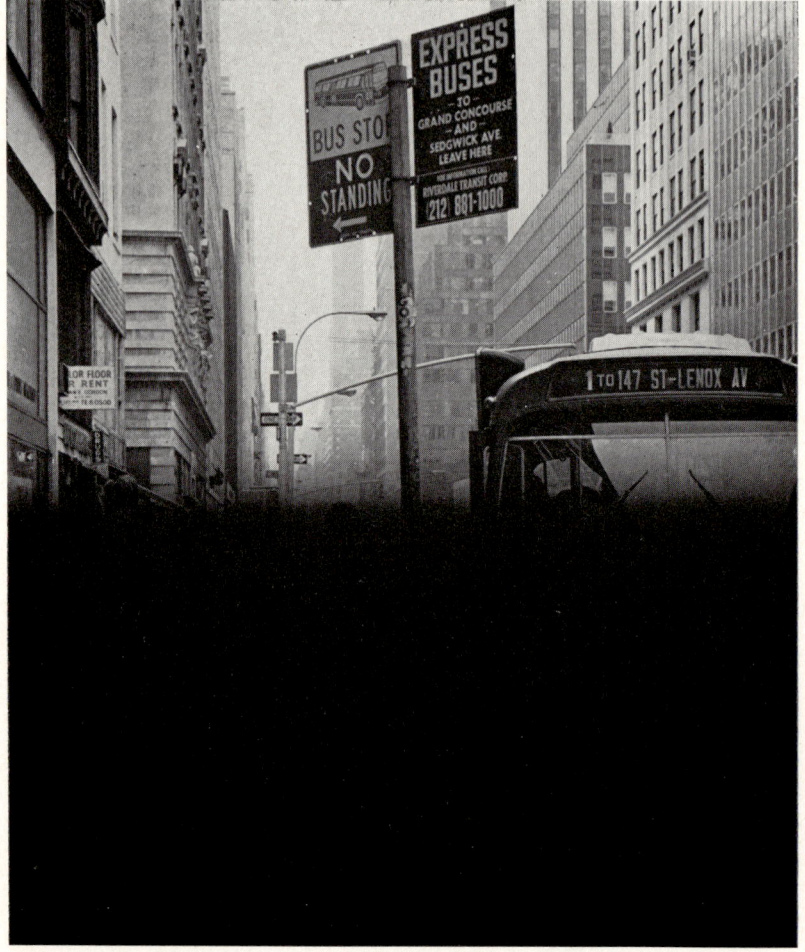

Figure XI-3. Inferior hemianopia interferes with mobility and reading.

used for the eye with better vision while awaiting resolution of the hemorrhages or uveitis.

Retinal photocoagulation techniques and vitreous surgery procedures offer hope for these patients.

It can be seen that an accurate diagnosis of visual loss is indispensible to the proper management of the partially sighted patient. It should be emphasized that the physician consulting in the low vision clinic may see patients whose diagnosis is not established.

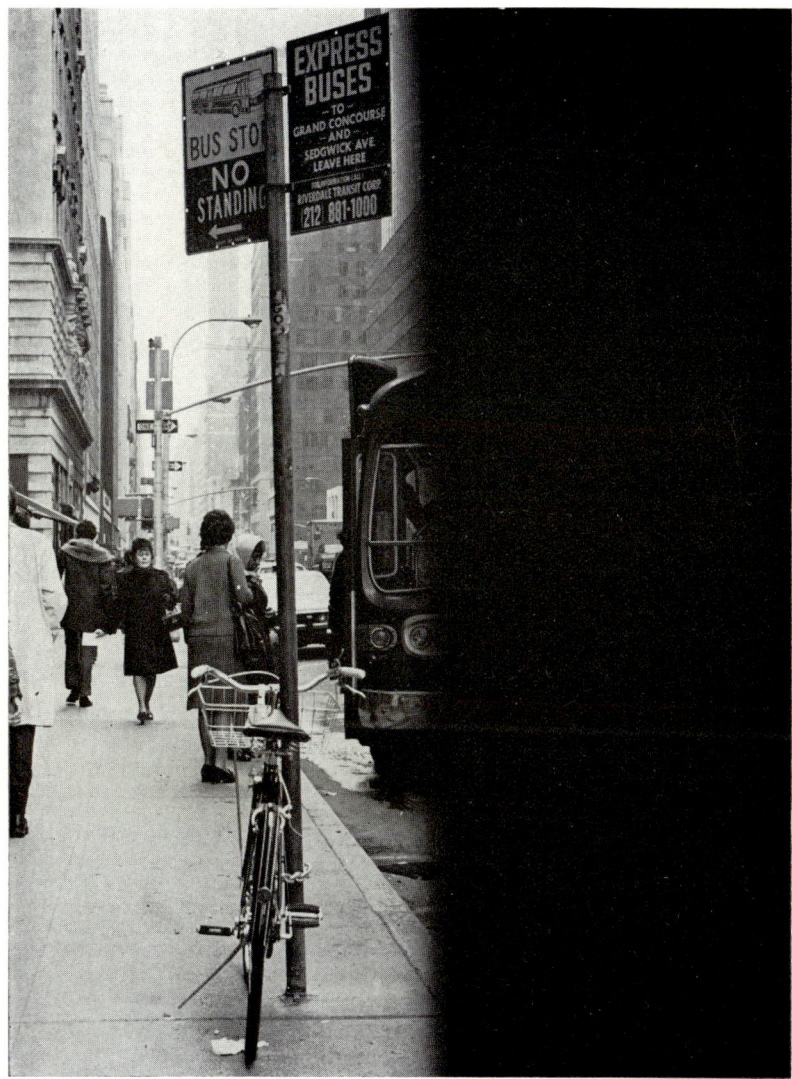

Figure XI-4. Right homonymous hemianopia interferes with reading from left to right.

Unexplained optic atrophy should be evaluated. Meningiomas, craniopharyngiomas, and aneurysms, (all treatable lesions) may present as progressive optic atrophy, and routine skull films may be negative. Further neuroradiological contrast studies are essential to ascertain the pathogenesis.

Motor disturbances such as unexplained nystagmus may be secondary to albinism, monochromatism, or tapeto-retinal disorders. Electroretinograms, electro-oculograms, and genetic histories are often necessary to establish the diagnosis.

The physician treating the patient with subnormal vision must always be alert to the possibility that ophthalmological or neurological, medical or surgical help is indicated to improve vision or preserve life.

· CHAPTER XII ·

Mirrors, Prisms, and Eccentric Field Defects

Wayne W. Hoeft

Introduction

THE LOW VISION patient with eccentric field restrictions is unaware of potential hazards in his normal surroundings, although he may move around fairly well. He may have 20/20 acuity but be more restricted by his field loss than a person with macular degeneration and 20/200 acuity. Any difficulties he may have are due to restricted peripheral fields, the field areas most necessary for mobility and the appreciation of moving objects. This article is intended to add to the low vision practitioner's storehouse of knowledge by offering suggestions which may help patients with eccentric field defects.

Consideration of Two Field Defects

Two types of defects will be considered. The first defect is hemianopic contractions which are normally chiasmal and postchiasmal lesions. Examples of causative factors would be tumors, trauma, and stroke. The second defect is a restricted peripheral field of 20° or less. This is a characteristic field defect due to retinal pathology in retinitis pigmentosa or to optic nerve atrophy in glaucoma.

Consideration of Three Field-widening Devices

There are three types of field-widening devices; mirrors, prisms, and reverse telescopes.

For hemianopias there are two possible optical means of solving the problem: mirrors and prisms. A right hemianopia is shown in Figure XII-1. For a patient with either a right or left hemianopia, a

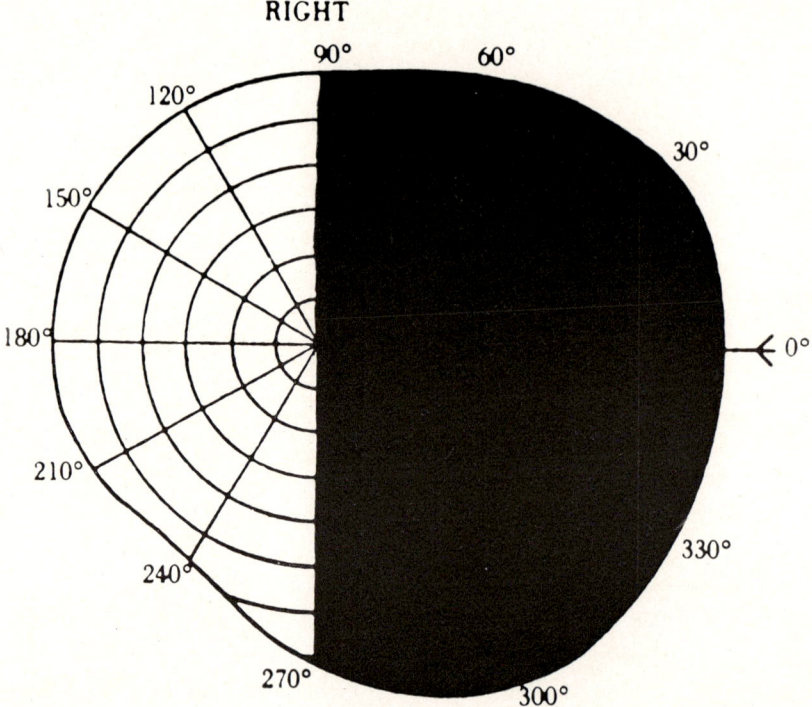

Figure XII-1. Right hemianopia.

mirror is placed in the good field of view, i.e. on the left for a right hemianopia. The patient would see a reversed image of the missing right field by turning his eye towards the mirror. With the second technique a 15-diopter prism is placed at the margin of the field loss with the base in the direction of the loss. By a slight movement of the eye in the direction of the loss, the patient looks through the knife edge of the prism. The image of the missing field moves towards the apex of the prism, or, in the case of a right hemianopia, to the left where it is seen by the functioning half of the retina.

For a peripheral field loss there are two possible approaches: reverse telescopes and prisms. A central field of less than 20° is shown in Figure XII-5. By reversing a telescope (Designs for Vision or Keeler), one would have a wider field of view but an image which appears farther away. Patients do not accept this method of solving

Mirrors, Prisms, and Eccentric Field Defects

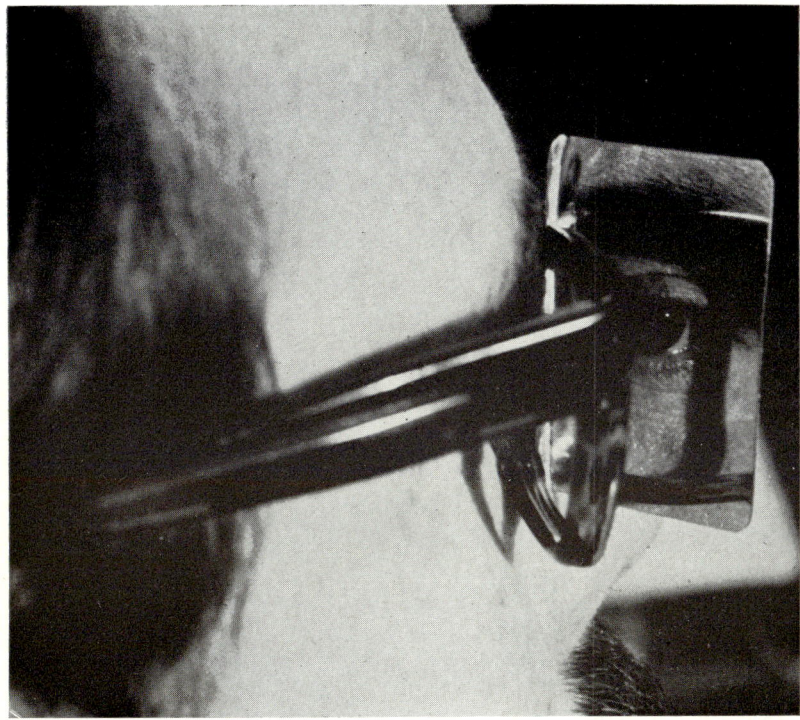

Figure XII-2. A patient with right hemianopia wears a mirror in the good left field. The image of the missing right field is reversed.

field restrictions because the minified image reduces the visual acuity which seems to cancel out the effect of the improved field.

In the alternate method of widening the field horizontally, two 15-diopter prisms are placed with their apices at the nasal and temporal borders of the field defect and their bases towards the field loss. These prisms may be applied to the carrier lenses of one or both eyes. By turning the eyes slightly in either horizontal direction, the effect of a larger peripheral field is obtained.

The cosmetic appearance of prescribed prisms must be considered at all times. In Figure XII-7 a front view of a hemianopic mirror is shown. Besides blocking out some of the normal field due to the mirror size and reversing the image, the mirror itself is quite obtrusive. Figure XII-6A and XII-6B show the front and top view

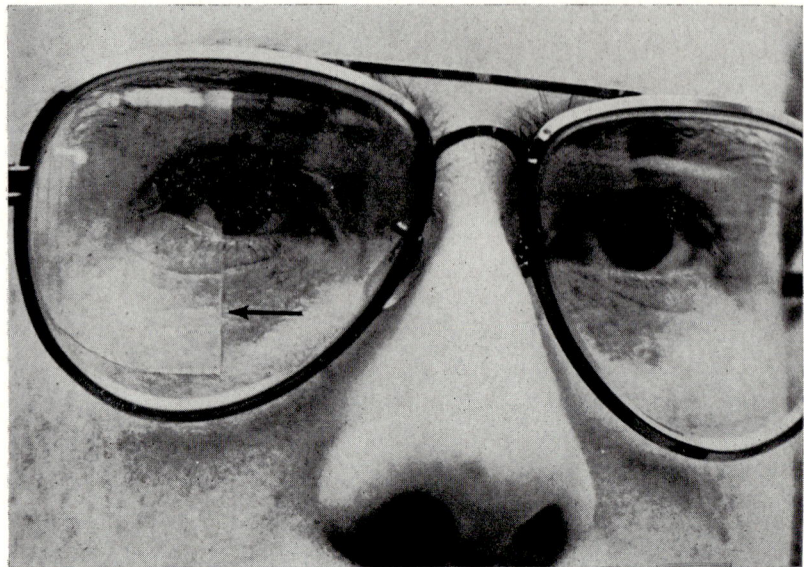

Figure XII-3. A Fresnel plastic prism applied to the carrier lens with its base in the direction of the field loss.

of a glass prism device for a retinitis pigmentosa case. The lens is quite heavy due to the weight of glass prisms, and if it is viewed from the top or side, it appears bulky. Will patients accept this aid? Some will, but experience shows that many will reject this aid on a cosmetic basis.

Press-on® Prism Techniques

A thin Fresnel prism made of plastic has been developed by Optical Sciences Group, Inc. The lens is called Press-on Optics by OSG and is carried by the major optical companies. This lens can be shaped to fit on the convex side of conventional glasses or a plano carrier lens. It is a practical, inexpensive way to demonstrate to the patient what the prism does to his field. If he cannot adjust to the lens and rejects it, the Press-on prism can be removed, used and reused indefinitely on any number of patients. The prism is hardly noticeable and therefore more acceptable to the patient. The lens is very light and solves a major objection to the glass lens, its weight. It can be drawn and cut to shape with ordinary scissors. The

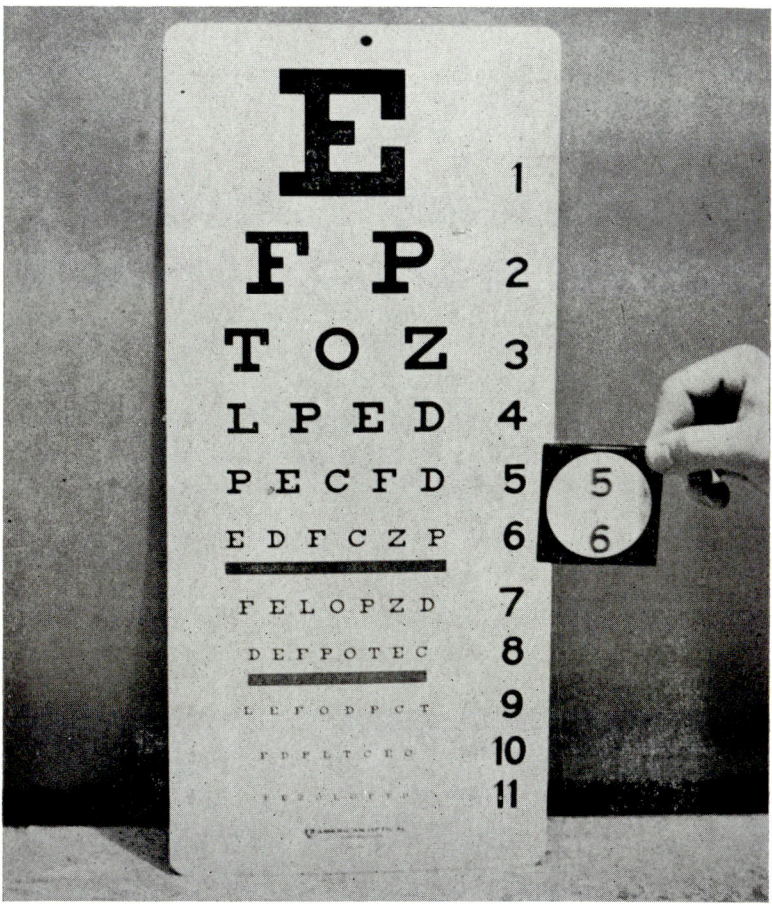

Figure XII-4. Demonstration of the movement of the field towards the apex of the Fresnel prism.

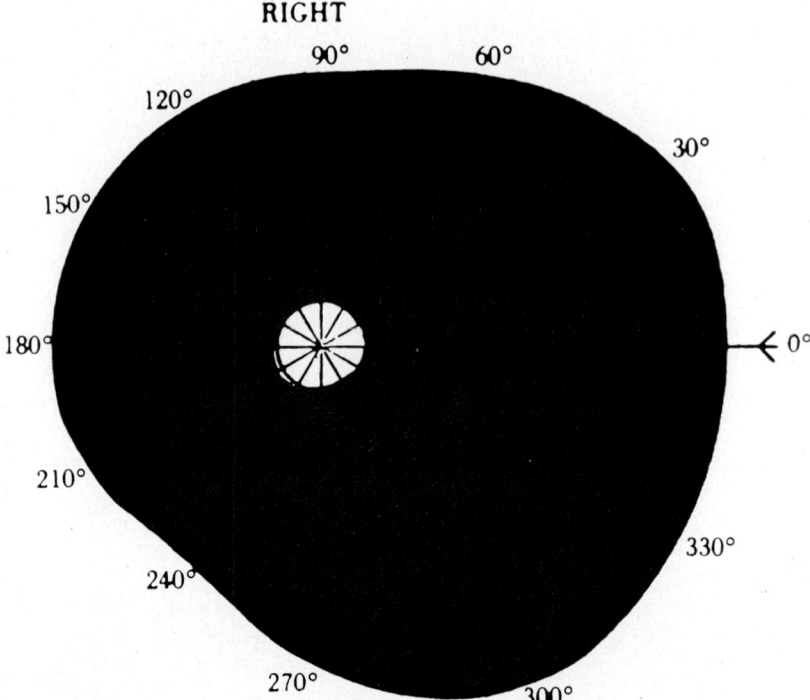

Figure XII-5. Restricted field of retinitis pigmentosa.

prism should be smaller in diameter than the lens on which it is to be mounted. It is easily cleaned with contact lens cleaning solution and can be applied to the front surface of the lens by immersing both prism and lens in water. The bubbles and water are pressed out before the lens dries. The Press-on prism can be easily removed and reapplied whenever and wherever required.

In applying prisms for hemianopias, one starts by placing the prism approximately 1 mm away from the pupil with the base in the direction of the field loss. For example, if the field loss is to the right, one places the prism on the right side of the lens 1 mm from the pupil with the base towards the right side (See Figure XII-3). The patient should be looking straight ahead. If the prism is not in the correct position at the clinical trial, it may be easily moved closer or farther away from the pupil. The best prism power, by experience, is

15 diopters. However, the patient may tolerate more or less depending on his particular case.

Eccentric field devices are probably more effective in cases in which the patient's perceptual abilities are still intact and motivation is high.

The patient with eccentric field defects gives the low vision practitioner his most interesting challenge in designing and prescribing unusual aids. Mirrors and prisms can be used creatively to help many people who are unusually motivated. As is the case with most optical aids, there is a drawback to their successful use. The patient must understand that he is in for many hours of special training in order to learn to tolerate the prism *jump* and the displacement of his environment. If he accepts this challenge, the practitioner may be able to design a mirror or prism system that can widen his world.

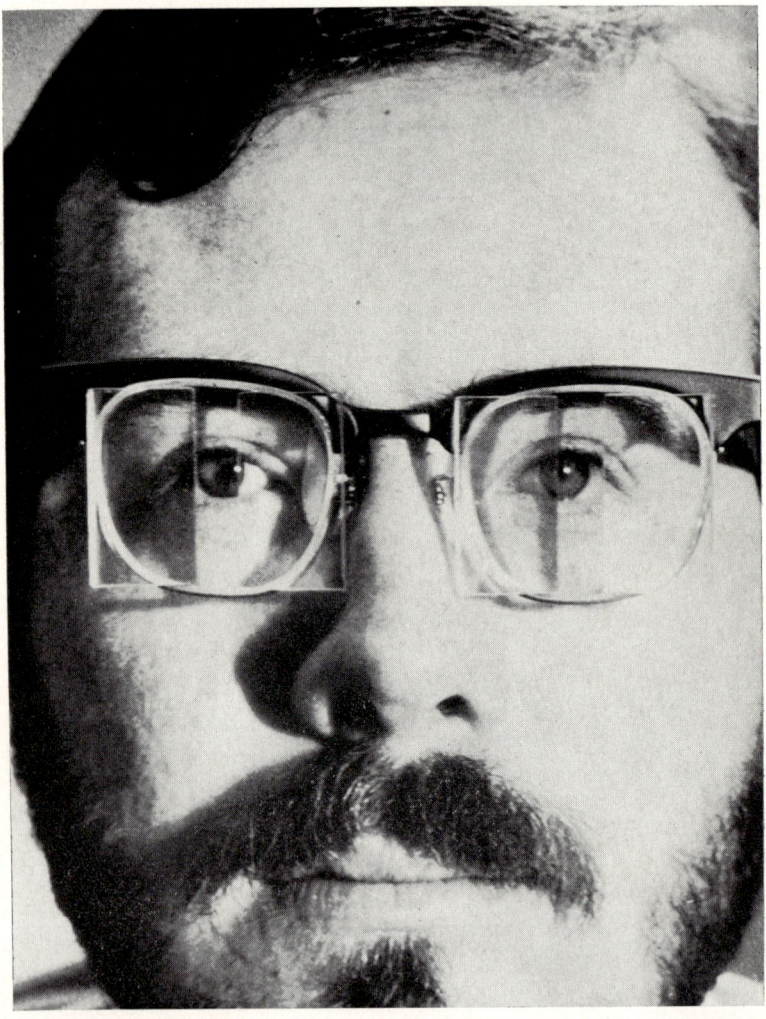

Figure XII-6A. Front view of a patient with retinitis pigmentosa wearing two 15-diopter prisms, base temporally and base nasally in front of each eye.

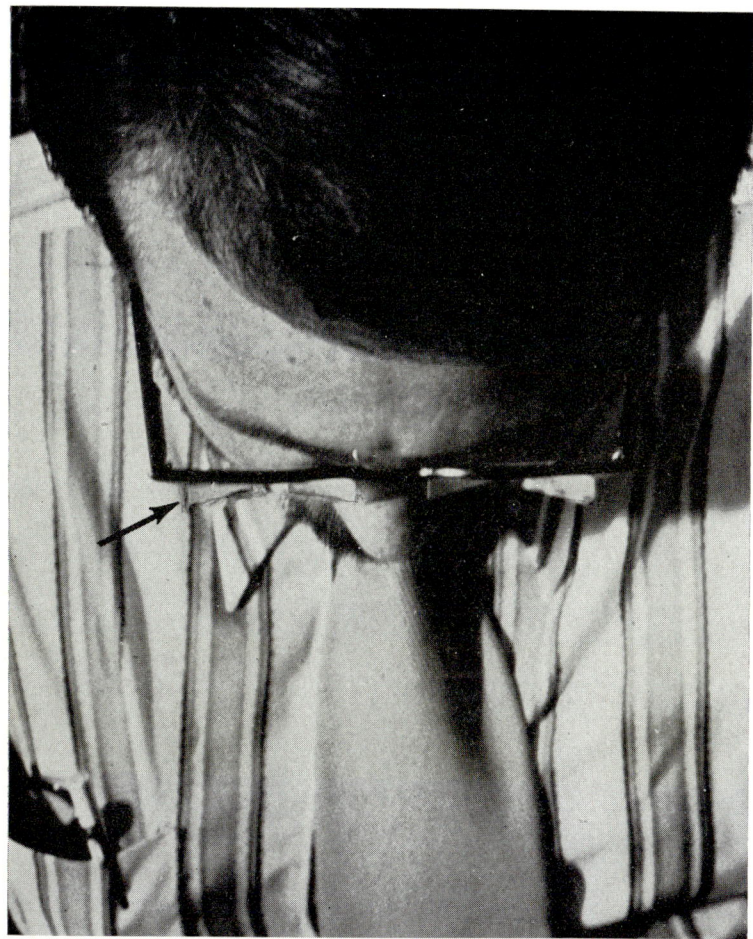

Figure XII-6B. Top view of the same case.

112 *Low Vision*

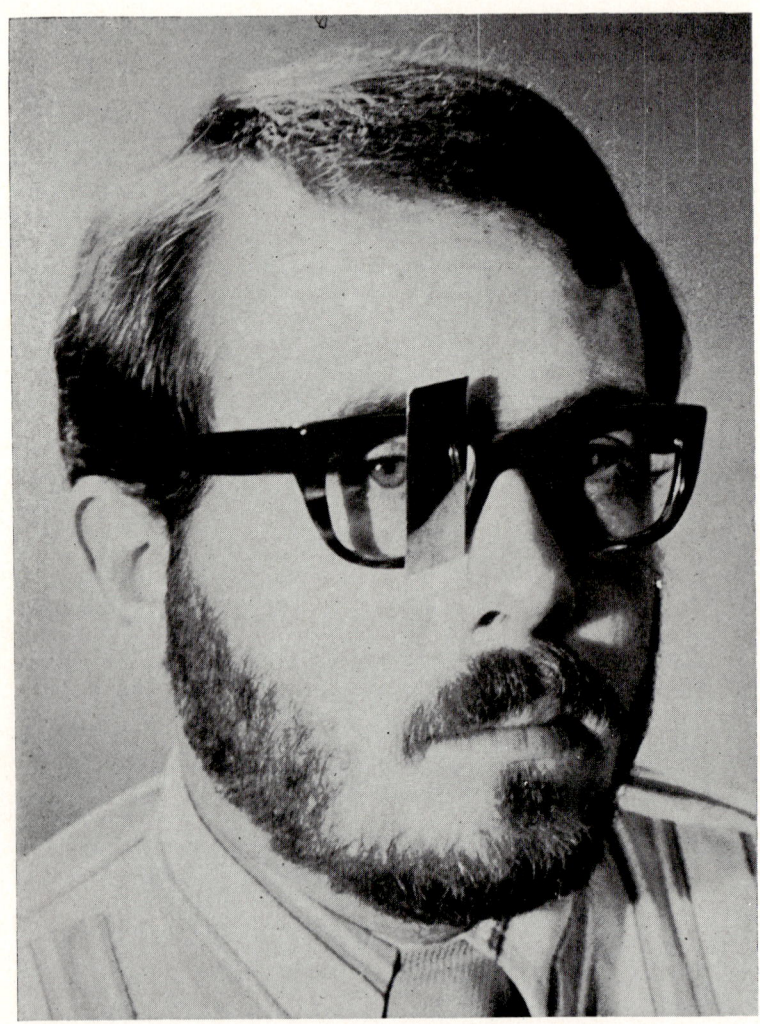

Figure XII-7. Front view of the hemianopic mirror demonstrates the poor cosmetic appearance of this device.

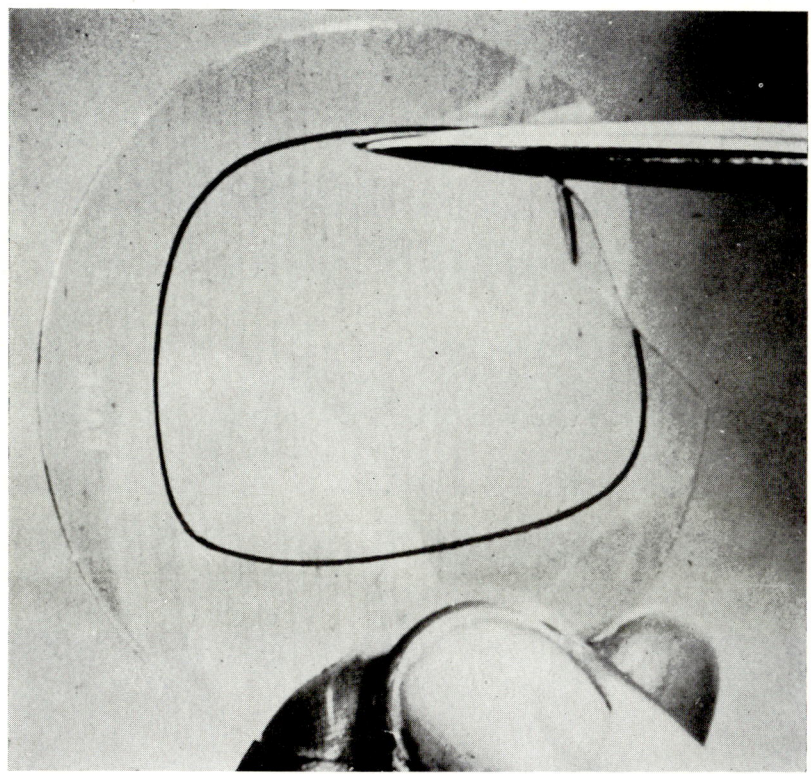

Figure XII-8. The plastic Fresnel prism may be cut to size and shape of any carrier lens.

· SECTION FIVE ·

Vision Rehabilitation from Childhood to the Vocational Years

· CHAPTER XIII ·
Pediatric Low Vision

Boyd H. Seidenberg

Introduction

THE GREAT majority of low vision pediatric patients have congenital ocular defects which may appear at any age from birth to adolescence. Trauma, infections, or neurological abnormalities acquired during the developing years make up the remainder of the cases.

A child's point of reference towards vision is different from that of the adult who has been visually educated and then loses his vision. The child with early vision loss cannot rely on visual clues and memories from a previously fully sighted existence. The child must become older before he fully realizes that he is different from others and that he functions at a competitive disadvantage. All these children, however, rely on their varying visual endowments for their everyday activities, for their education, and for their independence.

The clinician attempts to prescribe low vision devices which allow these children more effective use of their residual vision. Success with low vision aids in young children will depend much upon the parents' cooperation and their willingness to live with the visual prognosis for their child. It is, however, the pediatric patient himself who will be the practitioner's ultimate critic. He will not accept a useless aid, and barring physical defects or emotional attitudes, he will not reject a useful aid.

An optical or mechanical aid may make the difference between the child's education as a sighted or a nonsighted pupil. It is the responsibility of the practitioner to participate with parents, teachers, and social workers in educational planning for the patient. The following case report illustrates this point.

Case History

Case 1.

D. K., an eleven-year-old girl, was examined at the Lighthouse Low Vision Service in 1969. She was born with bilateral cataracts, underwent only partially successful surgery at an early age, and had a best corrected distance visual acuity of 3/200 in the right eye and 10/200 in the left. She read 12-point print with a plus 5 add. In order not to *strain* her eyes her education had been planned as though she were completely blind. Despite having a nonprogressive disorder, the school was teaching her braille. She complained that the braille was very difficult to learn.

At the Low Vision Service she was encouraged to use a 24-diopter lens for reading. This was an effective reading add of 11 diopters and allowed her to read 8-point print. Braille instruction was stopped. The patient was followed in the clinic for four years during which time her vision remained stable and she did well with the aid. At the age of fifteen she stopped using all spectacles because in her opinion they made no difference in her vision. The school started braille instruction again.

A revisit to the Low Vision Service revealed no essential change in her vision, and the school was once again asked to stop teaching her braille. The patient was referred for counseling.

The Low Vision History and Examination

A definitive medical explanation for the subnormal vision should be reached prior to the low vision examination. The general ocular and neurological examination usually requires extensive time and frequently utilizes sophisticated diagnostic tests. After these studies are completed a diagnosis or tentative diagnosis is reported. Those working with the child may use the diagnosis as a guide but not as a stereotype. A child should not be assigned to a category because of his diagnosis. Many diagnoses tell little about the capabilities of the child.

Inadequate school performance often initiates the referral of a visually limited child to a low vision service because the poor performance is blamed on the visual deficit. However, visual acuity and reading skills do not necessarily reflect each other. The ocular disease may not be responsible for poor achievement in the classroom. Learning disabilities in these children should not be overlooked. When a child with subnormal vision does not keep up academically with his visual peers, an educational evaluation is obtained.

In early childhood the visual state often cannot be determined with certainty. On occasion, a child will slip through the hands of more than one ophthalmologist by demonstrating a recorded visual acuity of light perception and later will show some useful vision. All partially sighted or *blind-labeled* children are candidates for a low vision evaluation and should continue to be followed as low vision patients as long as they have visual problems.

The low vision practitioner is often seen as a last resort. He should not be intimidated by the frequently impressive list of surgeons or institutions which have already examined the child. He is trained to keep an open mind when assessing the diagnosis and the visual acuity. He is primarily interested in finding a way to improve the visual function.

The low vision history should be as complete as possible and include all pertinent medical, ocular, behavioral, and school information. Reports of previous examinations should be available. Reports of teachers' observations of the child are extremely helpful. The parents must be asked to give an estimate of their child's visual function by a description of his activities. Ongoing medical or ocular therapy or planned ocular surgery may alter the visual outlook and must be given consideration.

The low vision examination begins with observing the child as he walks into the examining room. Is he led or does he walk with some assurance? Is he aware of the presence of other people, of lights, and of colorful walls? Does he walk with his head down, straight ahead, or turned?

Case Histories

Case 2.

E. B., a four-year-old, nonverbal, mentally retarded girl, had a history of being very difficult to examine and had never received correcting lenses. Her mother noted that the child held all objects very close to her eyes. The child appeared to have useful vision. A cycloplegic retinoscopy revealed a 5-diopter myopia in each eye. Glasses were prescribed, and on follow-up, the mother reported that the child never willingly removed the spectacles and functioned with greater visual awareness.

Case 3.

S. W., a 3½-year-old male, was referred to the Low Vision Service with a diagnosis of a "retinal pigment abnormality." No studies had been performed to substantiate the diagnosis. At the age of fifteen months he was noted to have a nystagmus and a to-and-fro motion of the head. A neurological evaluation was normal. The low vision examination revealed a mild pendular nystagmus and a left esotropia. The visual acuity was no better than 5/200. The ocular structures including the fundus appeared normal. A cycloplegic retinoscopy showed *8 diopters of myopia* in each eye. The child used the spectacles continually, and one month later the recorded visual acuity was at least 10/40.

Choosing the Aid

Once the information is assembled, the clinician must decide whether a special mechanical or optical aid would be of value to the patient. An aid should not be given for the sake of doing something. Some aids are too technical or complex for the child. Overprescribing may lead to patient rejection of all aids now and in the future. Considering the multitude of aids and combinations of aids available, some general guidelines based upon age groups and pathology are useful.

INFANTS AND PRESCHOOL CHILDREN. Infants and preschool children must receive the best refraction and spectacle correction as early as possible. This will help avoid the development of amblyopia. Unless aphakic, young children rarely require special aids for close work because of their ample lenticular accommodation. Aphakic children require a reading add.

> Case 4.
> A. G., a 4½-year-old girl, had bilateral congenital cataracts successfully operated upon at age one year. The parents reported that the surgeon advised against spectacles or contact lenses until age four. The uncorrected visual acuity was 4/200 which initially improved with an aphakic correction to 10/200, in six months to 10/50, and in one year to 20/60. The child is now performing well in a regular first grade class. Over the course of the year, the reading add was reduced as the vision improved, and she now can read 4-point print with an 8-diopter add.

PRIMARY GRADE CHILDREN. Children in the early primary grades usually have adequate accommodation to read the size print found in their textbooks. This is about 18-point print. For especially small print, such as is found in dictionaries at about the fourth grade level, a hand or stand magnifier is useful. If the child's poor visual acuity requires a reading add, this can be incorporated into a bifocal. Pediatric patients are particularly well suited to reading aids because they are accustomed to holding objects close to their eyes.[1]

Many children at this age appreciate a telescopic device for the blackboard. A commonly prescribed device is a 2.5x Selsi monocular on a neck cord.[2] When they sit in the classroom, they focus the device for the required distance and utilize it for a period of time without changing focus. A fixed focus telescopic device can also be mounted in the upper half of a spectacle lens and allows the child to see below the device for close work. A reading add may be prescribed as part of this lens system. There are many mechanical aids available to help the child with studying and homework. The obvious benefits of proper lighting and classroom seating should not be overlooked.

Case 5.

K. H., a ten-year-old girl in a regular fourth grade class, has congenital bilateral central chorioretinitis, and a corrected acuity of 20/100 in the better eye. She is bright, ambitious, and very cooperative. For the past two years she has used a 2.2x monocular Bioptic telescopic spectacle lens made by Designs for Vision.[2] She uses this for the blackboard and TV. It has a prefocused distance of 10 feet and yields an acuity of 10/50. For most print she uses no aid, but for mathematical fractions an 11-diopter hand magnifier is very useful.

TEENAGERS. Teenagers with subnormal vision frequently need reading aids in the form of a full spectacle, a bifocal, halfeye glasses, or a hand magnifier. It is usually not until the early teens that lenticular accommodation falls below 10 diopters. At that time an optical aid may be necessary for the first time. The highly myopic child may read through his minus lenses when young and remove them for increased magnification during adolescence. Telescopic devices remain useful for special purposes at this age. Contact lenses may be considered for distance correction.

Case 6.

V. B., a fifteen-year-old girl with congenital chorioretinitis and myopia, was initially seen at the Low Vision Service complaining of difficulty with blackboard vision. The corrected acuity was 10/100 O.U. She read the smallest print by removing her 4-diopter myopic correction. A 2.5x variable focus monocular was prescribed for the blackboard.

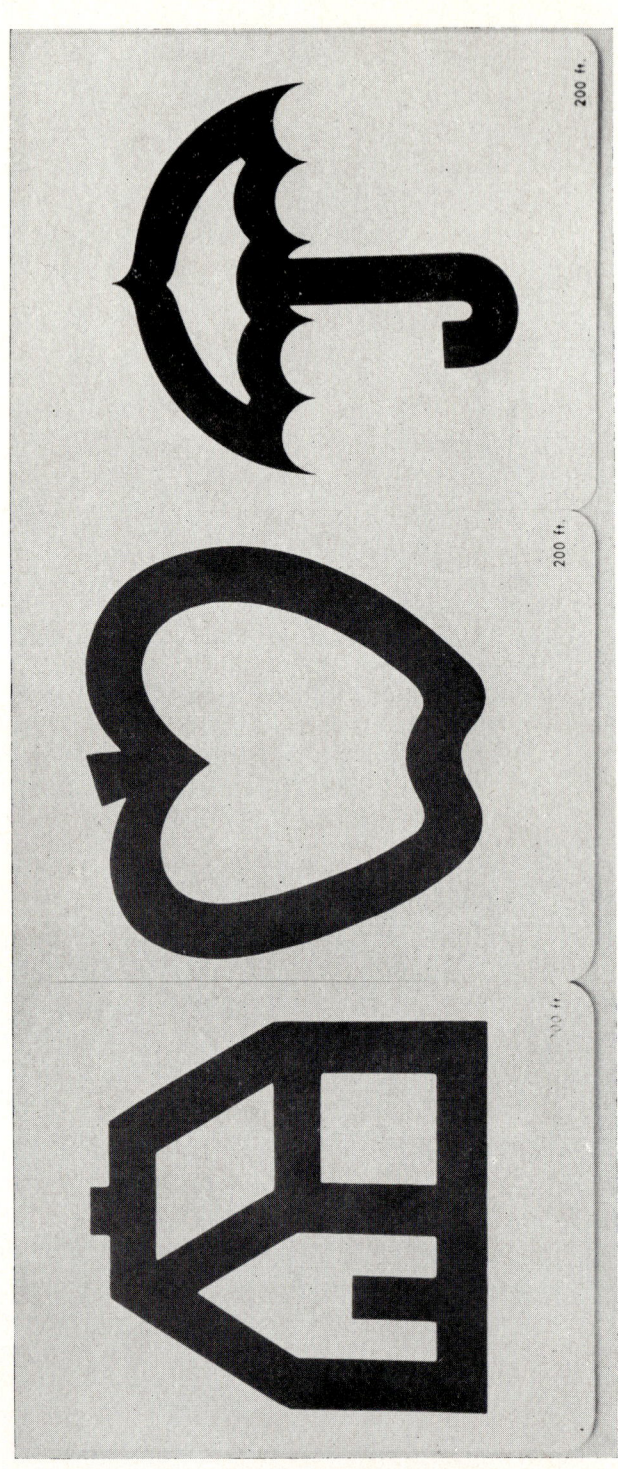

Figure XIII-1. Three symbols which are easily learned and more accurate than the *E* game. The flash cards shown are the *200* size. The range on the cards is to the 10-foot size.

During the next two years the myopia increased to 9 diopters. Near vision without correction remained stable, but she found it inconvenient to remove the glasses for reading. A 9-diopter bifocal add was given, and she has continued to do very well in school.

Determining Vision

Some children walk with their heads and eyes down to avoid ceiling lights. Others do so because of their fear of tripping, and others because they can see only nearby objects and have no reason to look straight ahead.

If a young child is carried by his parent, one should note whether his eyes move in the direction of objects which require visual appreciation or curiosity. When he enters the room, can he find the examination chair himself? After he is seated one should estimate his visual recognition of the silent paraphernalia around him. Does he reach for things close by or does he ignore them? One should note how he handles an object given to him. Does he immediately study it with his eyes or with his hands and face? Preliminary observations such as these frequently help determine which child is visually oriented.

The distance visual acuity of a child is important only if it has been accurately tested. If the child is older and cooperative, a reliable measurement is possible with a Snellen chart. A child who does not read letters is tested with the Lighthouse cards which employ the three symbols of a house, an apple, and an umbrella.[2] In each case the distance at which the test is performed should be ten feet or less. A nonverbal, deaf, or multiply handicapped child can be tested by matching pictures.

The vision of infants is estimated by rotating an optokinetic drum in front of their eyes. Lateral or following motion of the eyes indicates the presence of vision. The markings on the standard drum subtend the same angle as a 20/400 Snellen letter. If nothing else is available, a small flashlight is a simple method with which to elicit a visual response.

The near vision is determined with one of several reading cards which are either symbols or letters. The reading distance is recorded. All of these children take advantage of their high ocular accommodation for reading small print except those who are aphakic.

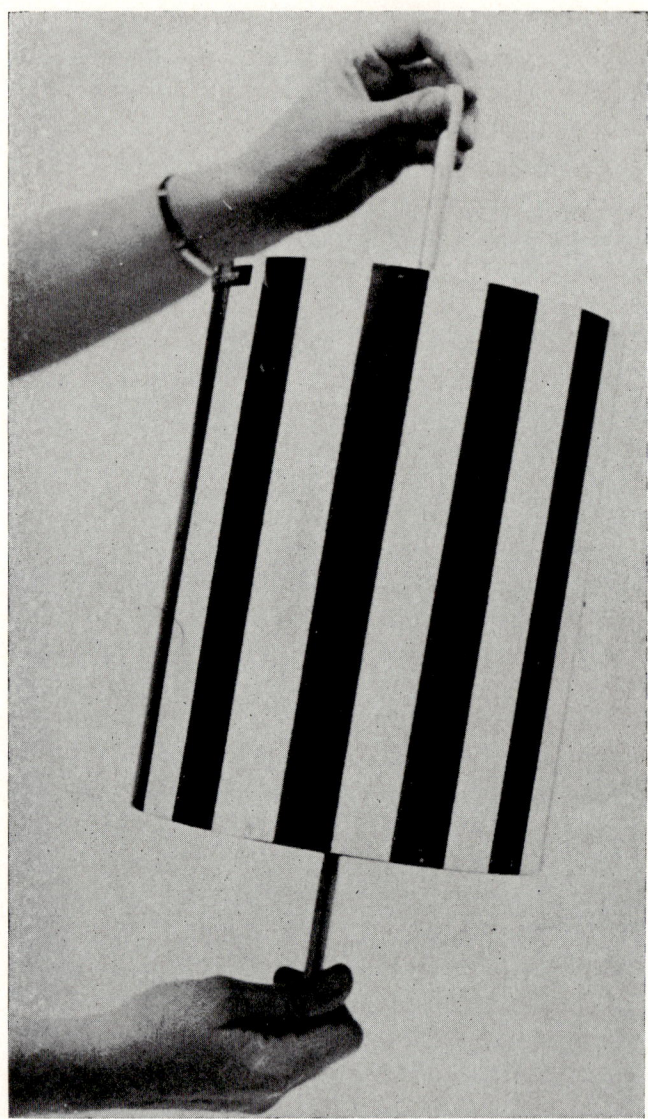

Figure XIII-2. Clinical evaluation of vision in infants or small children is estimated by rotating the optokinetic drum slowly counterclockwise and clockwise. Start at 5 feet and move towards the child until there is a response.

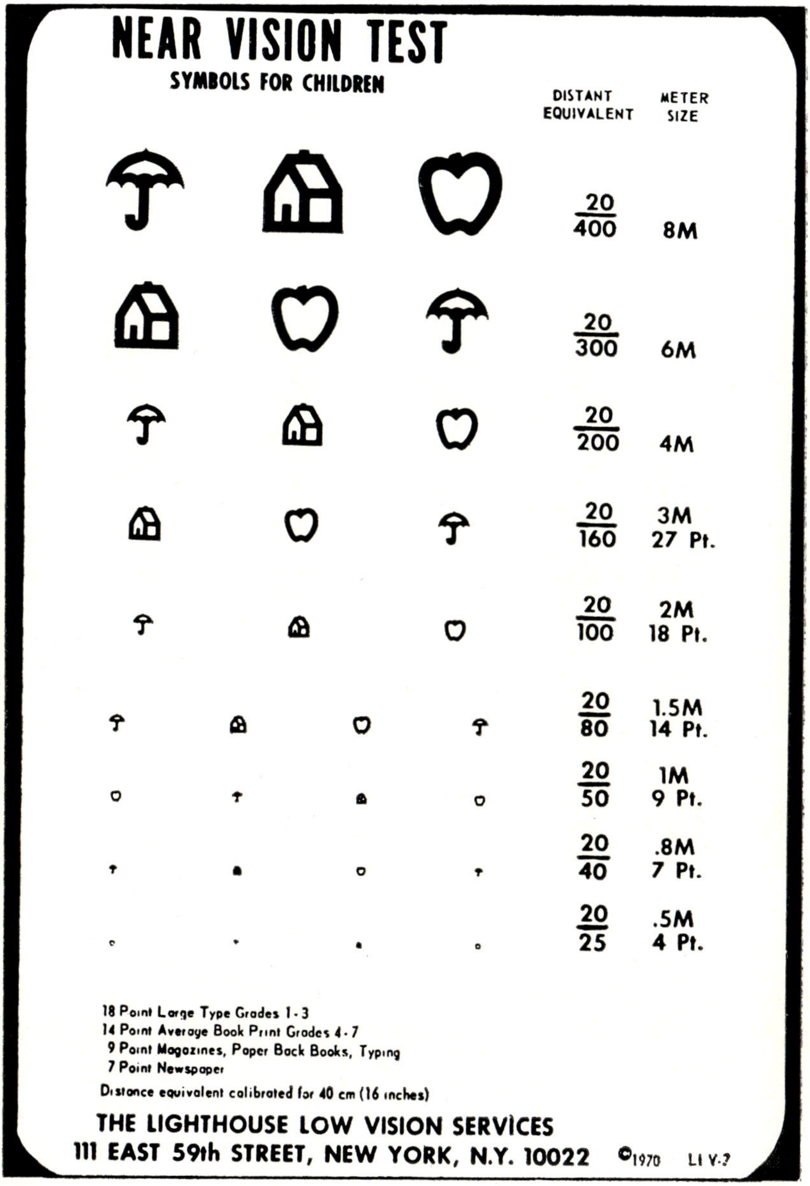

NEAR VISION TEST
SYMBOLS FOR CHILDREN

			DISTANT EQUIVALENT	METER SIZE
☂	🏠	🍎	20/400	8M
🏠	🍎	☂	20/300	6M
☂	🏠	🍎	20/200	4M
🏠	🍎	☂	20/160	3M / 27 Pt.
☂	🏠	🍎	20/100	2M / 18 Pt.
☂	🏠	🍎 ☂	20/80	1.5M / 14 Pt.
○	☂	▪ ○	20/50	1M / 9 Pt.
☂	▪	○ ☂	20/40	.8M / 7 Pt.
○	·	▪ ○	20/25	.5M / 4 Pt.

18 Point Large Type Grades 1-3
14 Point Average Book Print Grades 4-7
9 Point Magazines, Paper Back Books, Typing
7 Point Newspaper

Distance equivalent calibrated for 40 cm (16 inches)

THE LIGHTHOUSE LOW VISION SERVICES
111 EAST 59th STREET, NEW YORK, N.Y. 10022   ©1970   LI V-7

Figure XIII-3. A pocket-sized near vision card using reduced distance vision symbols allows useful near vision to be tested as early as twenty-seven months.

The examiner notes when a patient shifts his head or eyes to read. The child may naturally fixate with a parafoveal (or perifoveal) area when foveal vision is markedly decreased. He may also choose a position for his eyes and head which minimizes the effects of nystagmus.

A phoropter is not a good instrument for refracting the low vision child. Sometimes even a trial frame may not be satisfactory. Often the lenses must be hand held during the retinoscopy. A cycloplegic refraction should be performed every six to nine months for the young child with a high refractive error. In the past year I have seen several preschool children whose myopia had been severely undercorrected or undetected. Uniocular amblyopia is the most common type; however, a bilateral nonsuppressive amblyopia will occur when a clear image is not focused upon the retina of the young child.

Pediatric Eye Pathology

The ocular disorders most frequently encountered at the pediatric Low Vision Service from 1969 to 1972 are listed in Table XIII-I. A comparison with an earlier study (Table XIII-II) reveals some shifting of rank among the major groups. Some of the eye diseases which affect the low vision examination are described in the following pages with illustrative cases.

RETROLENTAL FIBROPLASIA: Retrolental fibroplasia is frequently associated with brain damage and learning disabilities,[4] and the child's schoolwork may be worse than his eyesight would indicate. The patient may be monocular. Myopia is frequently present. Some

TABLE XIII-I
INCIDENCE OF MAJOR PATHOLOGY (1969-72)

Age Group—Birth to Nineteen Years	
Rating	Diagnosis
1	Congenital Cataracts
2	Retrolental Fibroplasia
3	Pathology of the Optic Disc
4	Myopia
5	Macular Pathology
6	Glaucoma
7	Retinitis Pigmentosa
8	Optic Atrophy

TABLE XIII-II
INCIDENCE OF MAJOR PATHOLOGY (1953-68)

Age Group—Birth to Nineteen Years

Rating	Diagnosis
1	Retrolental Fibroplasia
2	Congenital Cataracts
3	Optic Atrophy
4	Albinism
5	Macular Pathology
6	Myopia
7	Glaucoma
8	Rod and Cone Defects

children reject the myopic correction by complaining that the lenses reduce the image size. One explanation for this is that the retinoscopy is not testing the eccentrically placed functioning macula. Many of the children do not require reading aids if they have sufficient myopia. They often use telescopes effectively for distance.

Case 7.

A.M., is an eight-year-old student in a regular class. The left eye has a very marked retrolental mass and no light perception. The right eye has a typical retinal fold. Bilateral nystagmus is present. At age three the recorded visual acuity was 20/200 O.D. At age four the acuity was 5/40 with a -20-diopter lens. At age six the child was functioning well in kindergarten with vision of 10/70 with the same lens. She could read 6-point print with the minus correction and 4-point print without correction. Most recently the recorded acuity was O.D. 10/50 + 2. With a 2.5x monocular she could read the 10/20 line. Regular size print could still be read with or without correction, and the distance lens had not changed.

ACHROMATOPSIA: Achromatopsia, a congenital condition due to the absence or abnormality of retinal cones, is diagnostically substantiated by an ERG. The basic low vision consideration is that vision is much improved in reduced illumination. Color vision is completely lacking in the complete form of the disorder. The treatment is provision of tinted lenses and shields that allow 10 to 20 percent light transmission.

Case 8.

J.D., a four-year-old student in the Lighthouse Child Development Program, had been followed by a local eye clinic, but a diagnosis had not been established. He was thought to have been born without vision.

Prior ocular examination reported normal eyes except for a nystagmus and an apparent lack of vision. The nursery school teacher at the Lighthouse noted that the child functioned better in reduced illumination than in the usually well lit school room. He was led to the examining room with his head down and his eyes closed. When the room illumination was decreased, he lifted his head, opened his eyes widely, and could maneuver around the room with relative ease. Trutone lenses with 20 percent light transmission had the same effect as lowering the illumination. By matching the Lighthouse symbols the vision was at least 4/100 on a first attempt. He was referred for retinal evaluation, and the consultant agreed with the diagnosis of achromatopsia.

ALBINISM: Albinism appears in the sex-linked ocular type or the autosomally inherited complete and incomplete types. The low vision considerations are similar in each group. Most have significant refractive errors. Although myopic astigmatism is probably most common, high degrees of hyperopia and myopia are seen. An impeccable cycloplegic refraction is a must. The child appreciates the full correction. Corrected vision is about 20/200. The presence of photophobia and difficulty with glare are variable. As a rule nystagmus is present. Many of these patients will do well with contact lenses. Coated lenses or tinted lenses to reduce glare are used when indicated.

Case 9.

A.G., was a seven-year-old girl with complete albinism. The best acuity was 10/100 O.U. with a high compound hyperopic correction. She read 12-point print with the distance glasses. The near vision was judged insufficient for her third grade level, and a plus 3 add in a bifocal was prescribed. This allowed her to read 4-point print. She did well with the bifocal during the follow-up period of seven years. Bright light was found to be an aid for her near vision. One of her frequent complaints was reduced vision when the spectacle frames went out of alignment.

APHAKIA FOLLOWING CONGENITAL CATARACT: In aphakia the visual acuity may be as good as 10/30 assuming no other serious ocular pathology. The result depends on the success of the surgery and on retinal involvement. A meticulous refraction is very important. The reading add should be prescribed as early as possible, and in selected cases, contact lenses are utilized. These children tolerate high reading adds very well.

Case 10.

R.L., a fourteen-year-old male born with bilateral cataracts, underwent cataract surgery at 1½ years. A bilateral pendular nystagmus is present. The corrected vision in each eye with a low compound hyperopic correction is O.D. 10/30−1, O.S. 10/70. The right pupil is very miotic, and the near vision is 14-point print at 70mm with a plus 4-diopter add. The patient is doing very well in school with the newly prescribed bifocal.

Conclusion

Several points are worthy of emphasis.
1. The visually handicapped child must receive a thorough medical evaluation aimed at discovering the correct diagnosis and visual prognosis.
2. Preschool children must receive the best spectacle correction as early in life as possible.
3. The low vision aids prescribed for children are related to their needs.
4. Subnormal vision alone is not the only explanation for academic failures.
5. Age and pathology may be helpful in determining the most useful low vision aids.
6. Success with a visual aid will depend largely upon its appropriateness and upon the support the child receives at home and in school.

REFERENCES

1. Sloan, L. L., and Habel, A.: Problems in prescribing reading aids for partially sighted children. *Am J Ophthalmol,* 75(6): 1023-35, 1973.
2. *Catalogue of Optical Aids* 3rd ed. rev.: New York, New York Lighthouse Low Vision Service, 1973.
3. Faye, Eleanor E.: *The Low Vision Patient.* New York, Grune and Stratton, 1970, p. 195.
4. Hoyt, William F.: Neuro-ophthalmological examination of infants and children. In Apt, Leonard (Ed.): *Diagnostic Procedures in Pediatric Ophthalmology.* Boston, Little, Brown, 1963, pp. 61-79.

· CHAPTER XIV ·

Psychological Evaluation of Low Vision Patients Using Closed Circuit Television

Robert J. Adrian

Introduction

THIS PAPER will focus on the closed circuit television (CCTV) and some of its implications for psychological testing. This presentation will report on procedures and findings utilizing the TV camera as an instrument which might have both psychological and cognitive implications. The utilization of the CCTV as an educational tool for the low vision person appears to have some promise as well as some drawbacks. First, the device gives low vision persons an opportunity to see visual stimuli at a more conventional reading distance. However, some clients resist the television aid because it is cumbersome and awkward to use. Second, the magnification of such visual material as printed or reading matter enables an observer to see a large projected image on a large screening field. The larger field becomes an important factor for persons with retinitis pigmentosa or other diseases which reduce the reading field. Third, the TV camera does require the person to master the complex skill of its operation, but the machine can be used at whatever rate is comfortable for the person. Figure ground difficulties are partially overcome since the figure can be either on a bright background or, when necessary, the background can be darkened by the flick of a switch.

Method

In order to determine if partially sighted individuals would show significant changes in terms of certain psychological test data, the following procedure was initiated. Seventeen subjects who varied widely in age but who were either candidates for vocational rehabilitation or in school were tested. All subjects had been referred for a low vision examination at the Lighthouse. Individuals selected had to have at least average intellectual capacity. Persons with known perceptual or other handicaps were not excluded.

Purpose

We wanted to determine if there was a significant difference in reading comprehension or reading speed when the subjects were tested both on and off the television. Our second interest was to see whether mathematical problem solving would show any significant change. We were interested in determining if the CCTV was more efficient than the prescription lenses or magnifying devices that had been prescribed.

Procedure

Each subject selected for study served as his own control. Subjects were exposed to the tests on or off the camera by random assignment. All of the subjects were encouraged to utilize whatever optical magnification devices they normally used. Subjects participating in this study represented eye diagnoses which involved (a) central loss and (b) peripheral loss. Accurate acuities with best correction for distance and near vision were taken before the subject was given any of the psychological tests. Low vision lenses were prescribed as needed to allow the person to read 1-M print. That is the comparison point at which the T. V. camera was set to provide the magnification needed for 1-M print during the test procedure. The visual acuities of the subjects were all under 20/200.

The subjects were given a brief habituation experience with the CCTV, and they rapidly learned to manipulate the controls. The examiner assisted the subjects in obtaining whatever magnification, light, and clarity they needed to perform the tasks. The subjects had the option of viewing the visual stimuli on either black on white or white on black, whichever was more comfortable for the subject. Ninety-five percent of the subjects preferred the white on black image.

Testing

The tests utilized in this study were as follows:
1. The Wide Range Achievement Test (WRAT).
2. The Bender Visual Motor Gestalt Test.
3. The Gray Oral Reading Test (Forms A & B).

The Wide Range Achievement Test was used as an initial screening base to determine the reading level of the subject prior to the administration of the Gray Oral Reading Test. Even though there is no alternate form for the WRAT, the plan was to analyze the test results on and off the CCTV. The arithmetic portion of testing also employed the arithmetic subtest of the WRAT. The possibility does exist that any differences in achievement between the pretesting and posttesting of the subjects (on or off the CCTV) may have been a function of previous exposure to the test items. Since these tests were presented to each subject in a random order, it is doubtful that this factor would influence the results to any appreciable extent.

The Bender Gestalt is a widely employed visual-motor-perceptual test. There was little difficulty in administering this test both on and off the camera.

The Gray Oral Reading Test had the advantage of having alternate forms comparable in difficulty and validity. Speed of response was timed by a stopwatch both on and off the camera. The set limit of ten minutes for the Wide Range Achievement Test on the mathematical subtest was also enforced. This time limit was adhered to both on and off the camera.

Results

The results to date indicate that the majority of the low vision cases evaluated on the CCTV did show positive changes on the tests administered to them. For example, in 75 percent of the cases the arithmetic scores on the WRAT increased by a mean change of four months when tested on the television. It would require a larger, more homogeneous sample of ages and visual diagnoses before one could determine if this change was statistically significant.

Only 15 percent of the clients failed to show any appreciable change in speed of reading on the CCTV or any increments in score on measures of reading comprehension. The remaining 85 percent of the subjects did show a positive gain both on the reading section of the WRAT and on the Gray Oral Reading Test. Speed of reading varied considerably, but those subjects who were unable to scan reading material off the screen showed marked improvement in scanning ability when they switched to the screen. It should be noted that scanning was not quantitatively but qualitatively evaluated; that is, observations of the subjects were made clinically, and it was noted whether or not the subject could pick up phrases and rapidly interpret the visual stimuli. Low vision clients with the diagnosis of retinitis pigmentosa showed the most improved visual functioning when utilizing the camera. Five individuals with progressive myopia showed striking changes in measured cognitive ability on camera. Two individuals who had been diagnosed as minimally brain damaged or as having a learning disability, and as demonstrating nystagmoid movements showed some improvement on the TV camera. However, these people had problems with line fixation which was equally distracting whether they were dealing with material on or off the camera. Doubtless this is due more to the central nervous system problems than to any visual factor. Two subjects diagnosed as albinos with field defects were able to use the camera quite satisfactorily but found the light emanating from the TV receiver very difficult to tolerate even for the relatively brief testing time required to complete the presented tasks.

It is important to note that 21 percent of the clients with field defects and high myopia were literally unable to utilize their vision off the camera despite any prescribed magnifying device. Thus, all of the data on these subjects was obtained from the TV camera. These persons were able to see individual words without the camera but with great discomfort and inaccuracy.

Additional CCTV Functions in Psychological Testing

The Low Vision clinic had been evaluating a number of multiply handicapped children, and the Lighthouse psychologists were particularly concerned about working with the ophthalmologists or optometrists to provide information on the possibility of organic perceptual problems. One of the tests involved in this study, the Bender Gestalt, could be useful in detecting visual-motor-perceptual problems. Frequently low vision children have not been able to respond to the Bender stimuli even with the aid of magnification devices. In several instances the Bender designs were successfully copied from the CCTV. Also, individuals reproducing the designs without the use of the camera would often produce records that were fragmentated, poorly integrated, and, in general, revealed signs of visual perceptual confusion. It was exciting to find that the Bender reproductions from the television screen improved appreciably and one could feel comfortable in ruling out visual motor problems in children suspected of having perceptual difficulties.

Another use of the CCTV that is beneficial in psychological evaluation of low vision clients is in the administration of nonverbal intelligence testing. Frequently low vision subjects do not have sufficient vision to be tested with performance on nonverbal test items. Thus, we are forced to use tests such as the Haptic Intelligence Scale or the Ohwacki. Both of these tests only have normative data for the adult blind (age sixteen and above). The former test only provides norms for the totally blind although the latter test does include norms for persons with partial vision. The camera has enabled psychologists to administer subtests of the performance scale of the Wechsler Intelligence Scale for Children (WISC) under the camera, and the children were able to perform some of the tasks when these subtests were used on camera. Despite the fact that the Kohs-Block Design Test contains chromatic stimuli and has to be presented as achromatic stimuli, it resulted in successful testing of these children. Administration of the Rorschach Ink Blot Test and the Thematic Apperception Test have also been successfully administered to subjects under the TV camera. The CCTV can provide psychologists working with low vision clients a valuable adjunctive tool in testing these individuals.

Case Histories of Adult Subjects

Two adult subjects evaluated with the TV camera may be of interest. These cases are clearly not typical but do illustrate the utility of the camera for persons in need of such a device.

The first individual was a forty-eight-year-old male with a diagnosis of retinitis pigmentosa. He had completely lost the ability to read ink print with any type of magnification. Pretesting without the TV camera was impossible for this person. His occupation required extensive work with numbers that he could no longer perform. The CCTV enabled him for the first time in two years to solve mathematical problems without assistance and with ease. The camera aided him to such an extent that he could read normal-sized print with average speed and excellent comprehension. It was an emotional experience to observe him looking at photographs of his children that he always carried with him but was unable to visualize until he had the assistance of the TV camera. His obvious need for the camera both vocationally and avocationally was clearly demonstrated and was the aid prescribed for this low vision client.

Another male subject, fifty-one years of age, also with a diagnosis of retinitis pigmentosa, was tested both with and without the TV camera. His reading comprehension and mathematical problem solving was superior even without the camera's aid. However, his reading speed was very slow and laborious without the CCTV. In addition, he experienced headaches when reading for a short period of time. When reading from the television screen, his reading comprehension did not substantially improve, but his speed of reading and scanning did improve.

With respect to our observations of persons with retinitis pigmentosa, it appears that the results obtained using the CCTV with individuals having peripheral field defects are significant.

Confirming our findings on cases of retinitis pigmentosa, Davis, Asarkof, and Tallman[1] have noted that two cases of retinitis pigmentosa had improved reading speed when using the camera. Also, research by Mehr, Frost, and Apple[2] has indicated that contrast polarity (white on black) has been found preferable for a large percentage of low vision clients using the CCTV.

Summary

This preliminary investigation reveals some positive preliminary findings. Although the sample presented to date is too small to be conclusive, statistical substantiation will be forthcoming on acquisition of a greater sample for analysis.

The TV camera obviously has value in a wide variety of problem solving, i.e. map reading, mathematics, musical note reading, and psychological testing. In the future it might be interesting to investigate CCTV as an experiential aid for young, preschool, visually limited children to help them identify and integrate concepts of environmental objects by presenting them as visual stimuli.

REFERENCES

1. Davis, P., Asarkof, J., and Tallman, C.: A closed circuit television system as a reading aid for visually handicapped persons. *The New Outlook for the Blind,* 67(3): 97-101, 1973.
2. Mehr, E. B., Frost, A. N., and Apple, L.: Experience with closed circuit television in the blind rehabilitation program of the Veterans Administration. *Am J Optom,* 50(6): 458-469, 1973.

· CHAPTER XV ·
Low Vision Patients In Vocational Rehabilitation Programs

Elisabeth Stern

Introduction

IN VOCATIONAL rehabilitation for persons with a visual defect, the emphasis is on the partially sighted, legally blind person who is pursuing vocational goals and who belongs to that broad age-group which makes up the labor force in general.

When visual function is so diminished that the individual is classified as *legally blind*, a number of rehabilitation services are usually required, one of which is low vision.

The success or failure of persons using optical aids depends as much on visual acuity and eye diagnosis as on expectation, age, general health, and intelligence. It is well known that a large range of visual acuity exists between 20/20 and 20/200 (legal blindness in New York State) and that variable amounts of useful vision can be between 20/200 and total blindness. In addition to the measurable acuity, there are such variables as field defects, impairment of color perception, and the general nature of the disease which caused the visual loss.

Vocational Rehabilitation Candidates

Observations in the past years have shown an increasing trend towards diseases which are not only affecting the eyes but which are of a systemic nature. These patients are not only visually disabled but are physically ill and often multiply handicapped. High on the list of systemic diseases is diabetes with its resulting retinopathy and other complications; vascular diseases which involve the eyes; neurological and postneurosurgical cases. Many patients are maintained on medications for the eye condition as well as for related and unrelated diseases. Although the drugs may be effective for the purpose for which they are prescribed, they often have side effects. Not feeling well, being drowsy, being nauseated, having blurred and changeable vision are added burdens to an already existing and serious disability. At best, it takes active participation, energy, and perseverance to adapt to special lenses. The anxiety brought about by the visual loss and possible further loss cannot be minimized.

Rehabilitation Candidate Subgroups

Within the broad group of the partially sighted, there are five subgroups of rehabilitation clients, from the person requiring single services to the multiply handicapped person who needs intensive, long-range services.

The first two groups are people who may be said to rehabilitate themselves. They tend not to be seen in formal rehabilitation programs. They may need a few selected single services. In the younger age-bracket are those with albinism, mild congenital optic atrophy, juvenile macular degeneration, and congenital cataracts. Under favorable circumstances they attend schools, sometimes special classes, and make the necessary adjustments without agency help. They are likely to be under the care of a private low vision practitioner or a low vision clinic and are likely to use optical aids effectively. The second group contains those adults who have already been established in professional or business life, who have either above average financial resources, or family backing, or exceptional professional qualities. They are less likely to require outside assistance. As in the previous group, they need help in the form of optical and nonoptical devices.

The third group is made up of people who are basically healthy and intact until their vision failure jeopardizes their job. They seek a few selective rehabilitation services and may need low vision aids. If these clients can be returned to their former position, this is obviously the best situation. They might also be retrained for a less visually demanding job in the same company.

In the next group are persons who are forced to abandon their careers, not because their visual function is so poor but because it has to be near perfect for their particular work; for example, where hazards are created by diminished vision (a machinist, a pharmacist, a transportation worker) or where the need for visual perception is paramount to the profession, (a fashion designer or decorator). Here every attempt is made to provide optical aids and training either to place these persons in an advisory capacity within their own particular field or to find an acceptable alternative.

A good number of clients belong in the fifth and last category. They are those who have the poorest remaining visual acuity and frequently the most complications in their lives. Many are also the physically impaired people who were mentioned before. Therefore they tend to be the most difficult and least successful candidates for using low vision aids. A realistic rehabilitation program takes into consideration the undeniable limitations some clients have in addition to their visual loss which, together with limited job opportunities, put gainful employment beyond their reach. They cannot achieve more than personal maintenance which in itself becomes a vocational goal.

Rehabilitation Procedures

Clients who come to The New York Association for the Blind for rehabilitation services are scheduled for a low vision evaluation provided they have some measurable vision. This includes exposure to recent innovations such as special telescopes and closed circuit television. Many are unaware that there is such a service available. Some are eager to get help, others are quite disinterested. This is often due to an inevitable degree of anger or depression or fear of jeopardizing the remaining vision. It is desirable that the client be evaluated for lenses before embarking on rehabilitation training. This allows him time to get used to the aid, and, with it, hopefully derive the most benefit from the instructional period. Some who initially reject help often become more amenable to a trial with lenses at a later date. Besides receiving counseling during the training program, they derive a great deal of support and encouragement from others who have similar problems solved by special lenses. Part of intelligent case management is the presentation of low vision in truthful terms to guard against overoptimism and unrealistic hopes by staff and clients. Otherwise disappointment and frustration may be expressed in rejection of lenses which do not restore *normal vision* and which may not be cosmetically acceptable to the client.

It is an accepted fact that the prescription of suitable lenses is not done on a one-shot visit. Clients are often seen several times before aids can be prescribed, especially in the early phase of the rehabilitation program. Once vocational goals are more clearly defined, a revisit may be indicated. One can then prescribe specific aids, spectacle, hand or stand magnifier, telescopic aid, or closed circuit television reader, to fit the actual work situation.

When a low vision aid has been prescribed, it is the practice at the New York Lighthouse Low Vision Clinic for a medical assistant to instruct the client in the use of the aid, to interpret the doctor's recommendation, and to work with the client's complaints, requests, and suggestions. The clients have an opportunity to ask questions about their eye conditions and medical problems. Suprisingly enough, many people do not understand their diseases and do not know how to take care of themselves. Without assuming the doctor's role, the staff can help to explain and clarify misconceptions. The importance of regular ophthalmological care is emphasized at this time.

Contact among staff in the rehabilitation department is designed to encourage the sharing of observations, the exchanging of recommendations, and the reinforcement of the use of prescribed near vision aids, telescopes, and tinted lenses.

Conclusion

In conclusion it should be said that visual aids may not be enough to fill the client's vocational needs but may be invaluable in giving him some measure of independence in his private life. He may have to function mainly with nonsighted techniques in his work and in his home, but he may be able to spot-read or do some occasional viewing. Likewise, telescopic aids should be considered not only for mobility purposes but for their place in recreational pursuits where they can afford a great deal of pleasure.

It is worthwhile for the individual who will appreciate it, to improve what vision there is by whatever means it can be improved.

· CHAPTER XVI ·

Rehabilitation Using Aids Modification During Vocational Training

KAY McDONALD

In its broadest definition, we speak of rehabilitation as the restoration of the handicapped person to the fullest mental, physical, emotional, social, vocational, and economic usefulness of which he is capable. To this end the vocational rehabilitation counselor often finds himself joining with others in a search for ways and means of helping a person work towards that restoration. Part of the broad program of rehabilitation includes the investigation of optical and visual aids.

Diagnostic Phase of Rehabilitation

There are basically four phases to The Lighthouse program: diagnostic, prevocational or personal adjustment, vocational and placement. During the diagnostic period, those clients with any degree of residual vision are given a low vision examination to determine their abilities in such areas as mobility, personal management, manual arts, and communication skills. For the homemaker, this examination might result in a prescription for a simple hand magnifier to help her read the labels on a food can; for the student, a monocular or binocular aid to help with blackboard work, films, and other visual materials; for the typist, a telescopic lens to help bring the copy up closer.

A client came to the rehab counselor's office in an excited state. He had been to the Low Vision Clinic the day before for the first time and was given an Ary loupe that he could wear over his glasses. He had lost a substantial amount of sight within the year and had been quite depressed over his restricted activities. He had difficulty visualizing measurements and design plans for his hobby which was making cabinets and other small furniture pieces. A click ruler and the clip-on loupe over his glasses were the necessary instruments to get him started again.

Another client, a woman, arrived in an equally excited state and said that her hand magnifier was a big help. Now she could go to the supermarket and read prices on food items. For that woman, reading the food prices was a major accomplishment full of happy meaning.

In the total rehabilitation process, then, visual rehabilitation through low vision aids is often the first step in the ongoing rehabilitation process. Because a person's needs, objectives, and environments are forever changing, visual aids must be continually adapted to meet these changes.

Rehabilitative Aids Adaptation

In the process of rehabilitation, we recognize that clients do not respond predictably to what is offered. Workers in rehabilitation are familiar with the type of client who accepts his aids with little or no difficulty.

But just as familiar is the *marginal* person, the individual who rejects the aid outright or is too depressed or too disturbed to be interested in the limited help the aid can give him.

What, for example, makes the man with 5/200 vision and field defects function better than a man with 20/200 vision and no field defects? What makes a dependent person fearful of the independence an aid might give him? The reasons for rejections of the aid are complex and varied and often require help from the counselor or other members of the rehabilitation staff in guiding the client towards understanding his attitudes. The following case history is of a client who accepted aids and used them to their maximum potential.

> Susan was a young woman of twenty-six when she developed bilateral macular scotomas due to neurological disease. It was a depressing and confusing time for Susan which was not improved by various visits to ophthalmologists who seemed to be unfamiliar with available rehabilitation services. It was not until two years later that her current ophthalnologist, her fourth, sent her to the rehabilitation agency. Prior to the neurological onset which decreased her vision to the point of legal

blindness she had worn glasses for myopia. When she first realized she had lost some vision, she was given a pair of glasses with magnification for reading. She also used a 6x and a 10x hand magnifier for spot-reading. As her needs changed visually and educationally with her entrance into graduate school, she changed to the same prescription in a half-eye frame. This had the advantage of allowing her to read and to see her surrounding environment without the distortion from the upper part of a reading lens. It soon became apparent, however, that her distance vision was not that good, and she was not really profiting any longer from the advantages of a half frame. That was the point at which she started to wear a pair of 10x full-vision glasses. The client, however, did not complete graduate school by simply relying on low vision aids. The use of reader services, large print material, books on tapes, and felt-tipped pens were also an important factor in getting through the large amount of reading material. The reading aids provided her with the freedom to cover such selective materials as bibliography lists, outlines, and library catalogues at times when readers were not available or time did not permit the tedious search through taped material. An important nonacademic use for an optical aid was its function for personal reading material such as a letter from a department adviser at school, a bank statement, or a postcard from a friend.

Two additional aids which were also of great help to the client on a personal level included a Selsi 2.5x monocular aid for television and a Selsi 10x monocular which she used for reading street signs and numbers on buildings.

In the classroom, some of Susan's work involved films, field trips, and medical demonstrations, all of which required distance vision. She was greatly helped by a good pair of Selsi 6x binoculars. The same binoculars were used in her social life to make the theater, the ballet, and the movies a more pleasurable experience.

When she began working in her job as a social worker, helping a client fill out forms became a problem. A pair of half-eye lenses was again prescribed to allow her to write straight on a line and to see the client at the same time.

This client's experience underscores some basic points: (a) the emphasis is on the optimum use of residual vision; (b) visual rehabilitation is often an ongoing process; (c) a person's optical needs must be tailored to his mobility, homemaking, social, educational, or vocational needs; (d) continued correction, modification, and refinement of the lens is often necessary for the successful implementation of a person's rehabilitation goals; and (e) a person learns more about types of optical aids and what they can do for him as he progresses in the program.

The latter point is one in which the rehabilitation counselor sees the necessity for close contact with the low vision clinic or for what Doctors Jose and Springer[1] in their article on low vision aids and the interdisciplinary approach call the need for "cooperation and communicating."

Continuing Rehabilitation

The usual practice in a rehabilitation program for the visually handicapped is to see at the beginning of the diagnostic period those individuals with any degree of vision. At this point, optical aids are often prescribed. However, some counselors feel that it may be premature to give aids on the first visit; the client may need a complete diagnostic evaluation before the visual needs can be fully understood. As the client's program progresses, new problems may arise requiring further modification and refinement of the person's aids. Since the counselor sees the client more frequently, he should bring new developments back to the low vision staff for a fuller interpretation of the client's visual needs based upon the observations of all staff members during the evaluation period. This, for example, often happens in mobility. A client and his instructor may see things as they progress through the diagnostic period that were not apparent at the beginning of instruction.

Without frequent follow-up visits, some clients can become easily discouraged with their aids. More training for the client in the use of aids is another area in which the low vision clinic plays an active role. Many times a client gives up if he has not been taught to use an aid or what to expect from it.

If the vision is adequate and the aid appropriately prescribed, extra training will be beneficial. Many times the client *cannot* use an aid as predicted because of the nature of his eye disease. The counselor should be sensitive to a natural tendency on the part of the client and staff to force the use of aids in every case in which there is partial sight. Then a rehabilitation counselor working closely with a low vision expert may have to change the program to include other kinds of nonvisual aids.

There is no question that the low vision clinic has made an enormous contribution to the field of rehabilitation in a facility that serves visually limited individuals. No one knows better than the client the joy of being given increased vision through an optical aid. To be able to read a letter from a friend, however haltingly, to balance a checkbook, or to watch a favorite TV show are moments in that person's life which cannot be measured by statistics or captured in a professional's report. They are the stuff of which rehabilitation is made, the restoration of which it speaks.

REFERENCE

1. Jose, R. T., Springer, D.: Optical aids: an interdisciplinary prescription. *The New Outlook, 67*:12-18, 1973.

· CHAPTER XVII ·
Cases in Which Optical Aids Made A Crucial Difference

George O. Hellinger

Introduction

Within the past twenty years a virtual revolution has taken place in the rehabilitation of the partially sighted person. There has been a progressive acknowledgement of the value of vision, even though impaired. New attitudes in this area have allowed more acceptance of the value of low vision aids. Patients with partial sight now have a choice of many devices or aids to help them make the best use of their vision.

The approach in this new era is to recommend several aids: a telescope for distance, microscopic spectacles for near work, and, of course, the mainstay of simple spectacle corrections. Absorptive lenses are also an important challenge in prescribing for certain eye conditions. In addition to the technical considerations in prescribing, factors such as motivation, personality, and general intelligence must be considered by the examiner.

As in any rehabilitation process, the concept is to stress ability rather than disability and to emphasize gains that may be small but meaningful.

Case Histories

The following cases show examples of the many factors involved in prescribing for patients who have complex needs and problems.

Case 1.
   Patient: C.A., rehabilitation counselor, first seen in 1970 at age twenty-three.
   Condition: macular degeneration, O.U.

Cases In Which Optical Aids Made A Crucial Difference 147

Distance Visual Acuity:
  without correction, 10/200 O.U.
  with correction, 10/100 O.U.
  absorptive lenses.
  color—grey.
  absorption—88 percent.

This first case is an excellent example of the importance of reducing illumination in some cases where there is marked cone dysfunction. Highly absorptive dark lenses are used for these cases of central loss; for example, in macular degeneration, central cataracts, and corneal involvement in which stimulation of rod function is the primary goal, these lenses allow only 10 percent transmission, and the special frames eliminate all the light from the sides. Not all patients with macular lesions will respond to this degree of absorption of light, particularly if they still have some cone function. These patients often accept 60 percent gray absorptive lenses. This case also shows what variety of aids are necessary to maintain this young man in his job.

Other Aids Prescribed:
1. hand magnifier, 7x.
2. 8x microscope, 6-point type.
3. 10x hand-held prism monocular telescope for viewing street and bus signs.

Case 2.
Patient: B.W., first seen in 1968 at age five (now age eleven).
Condition: retrolental fibroplasia O.U.
Distance Visual Acuity: 5/200 OD, light perception, OS.

This patient stresses the importance of several visits to establish rapport and proper motivation.

An overactive problem child who was considered uneducable and a candidate for a school for the blind, low vision aids made it possible for him to enter a school for normal children, and to maintain his status there.

Although very slow to accept any optical aids, an inconspicuous 3.5x ring telescope encouraged him to try other optical aids.

Aids Prescribed:
1. microscopic spectacle, 8x. He is able to read 4-point type.

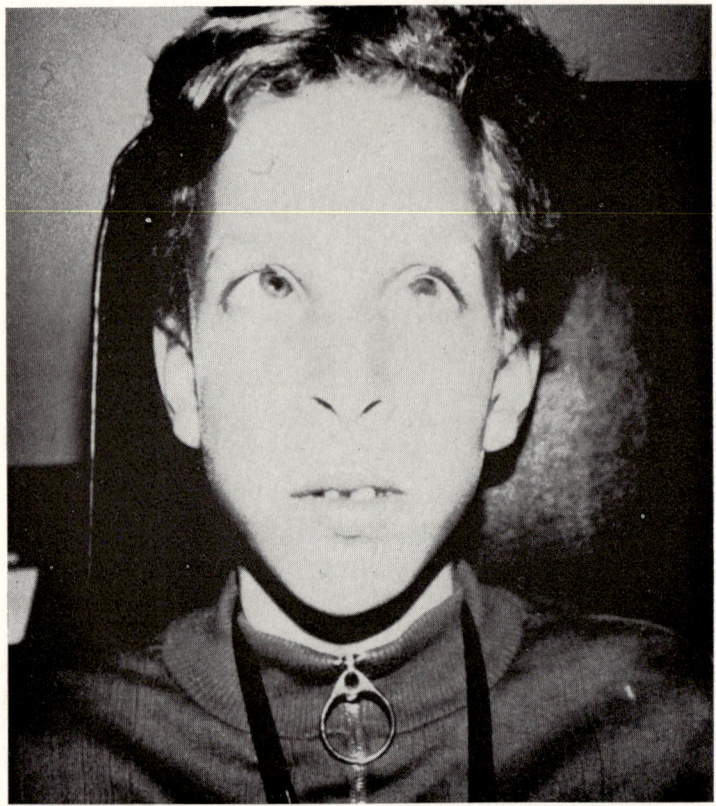

Figure XVII-1. This boy with R.L.F. needed many visits, reassurance, and training to use optical aids successfully. Vision was 5/200 OD, LP, OS.

    2. 1.7x telescopic spectacle for television.
    3. 1.7x telescopic spectacle with a $+2$ cap for music and drawing.
    4. 6x wide angle monocular telescope.

Case 3.
Patient: A.P., first seen in 1961 at age thirteen (now age twenty-five).
Condition: microphthalmos, O.U.
Distance Visual Acuity:
  Without correction: 10/350 OD.
                        LP OS
  With correction: 10/160 OD
                        LP OS

This young man completed his master's program in business ad-

Cases In Which Optical Aids Made A Crucial Difference 149

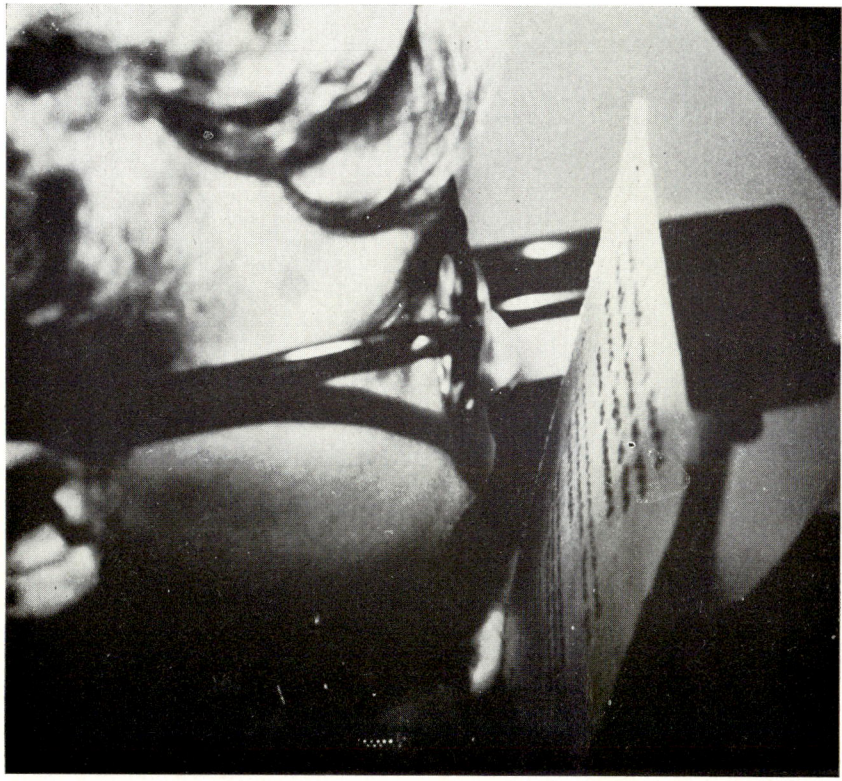

Figure XVII-2. Reading 4-point type with an 8x microscopic spectacle.

ministration. He is an excellent mechanic and student of electronics. He built his own closed circuit television with impressive innovations.

A high add bifocal may be prescribed for the patient who has always worn bifocals, who has a significant refractive error (an aphakic patient for example), or who finds them more convenient for a job as in this case.

Aids Prescribed:
    1. Photogray® spectacles.
    2. high add, + 16.00 bifocals which enable him to read 6-point type.
    3. 8x microscopic spectacles which enable him to read 4-point type.
    4. ring telescope, 3.5x.

Case 4.
Patient: J.Y., first seen in 1968 at age forty-five.

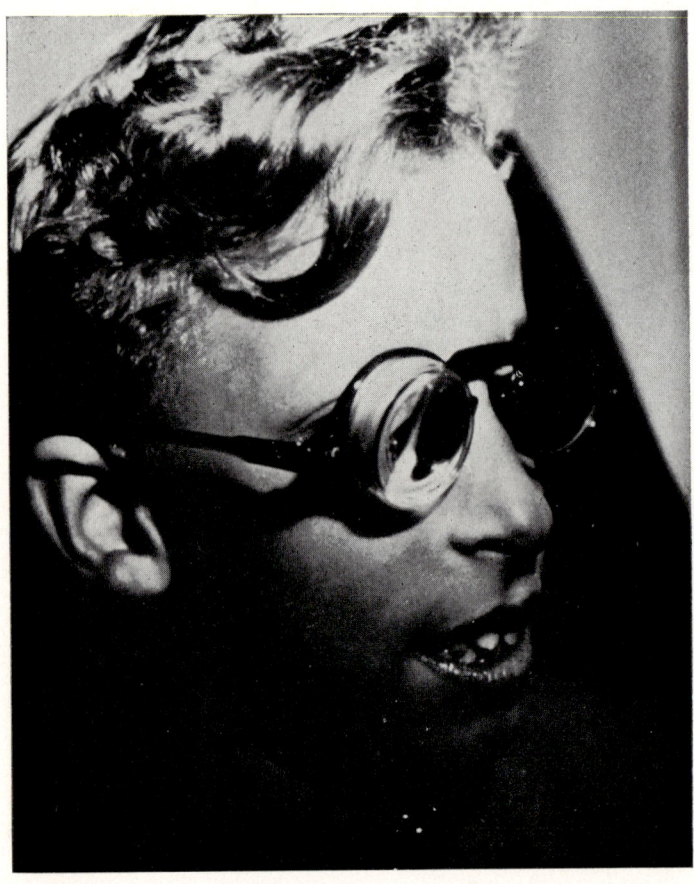

Figure XVII-3. Using a 1.7x full-diameter telescope to watch television.

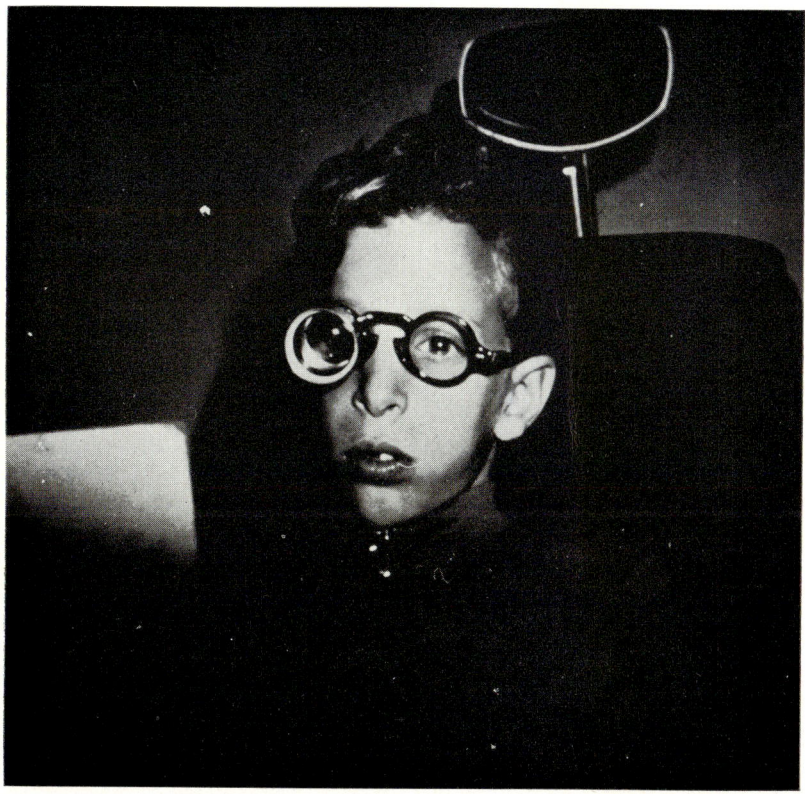

Figure XVII-4. A 1.7x telescope with +2.00 cap gives him intermediate range for music and drawing.

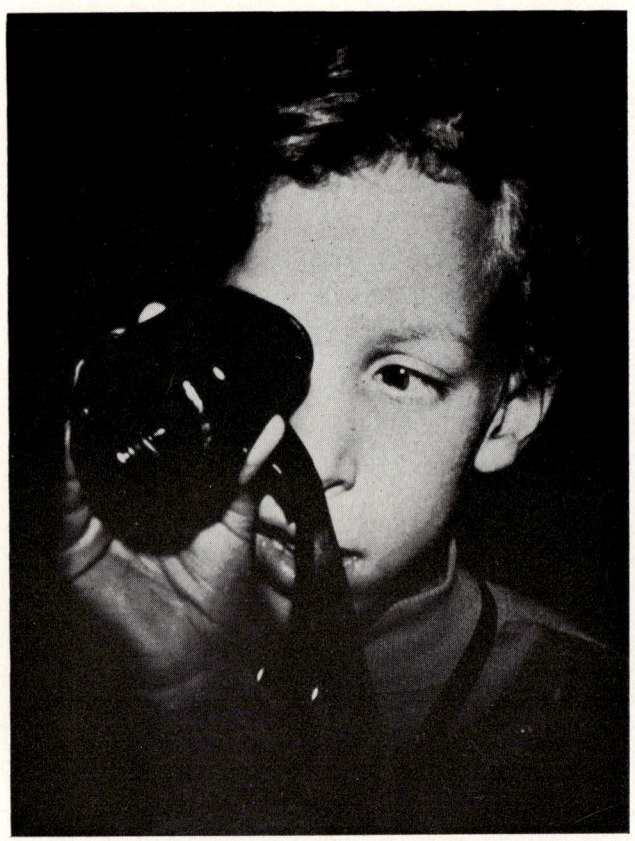
Figure XVII-5. Using a 6x monocular telescope for far distance.

Cases In Which Optical Aids Made A Crucial Difference

Condition: toxic amblyopia, O.U.
Distance Visual Acuity:
  20/300 O.U. without correction.
  20/200 O.U. with correction.

This case is an example of perseverence on the part of the examiner and patient. Here was an attorney with definitely unrealistic goals. However, counseling, encouragement, and guidance (plus low vision aids) permitted him to establish himself in a business which used to be his hobby.

Aids Prescribed:
  1. absorptive bifocals add +6.00 O.U. for constant wear.
     color—gray.
     absorption—20 percent.
  2. absorptive bifocals add +6.00 O.U.
     color—gray.
     absorption—30 percent.
  3. 3.5x telemicroscopic spectacle with 16 in working distance for his occupation.
  4. 6x30 binocular for the theatre and travel.

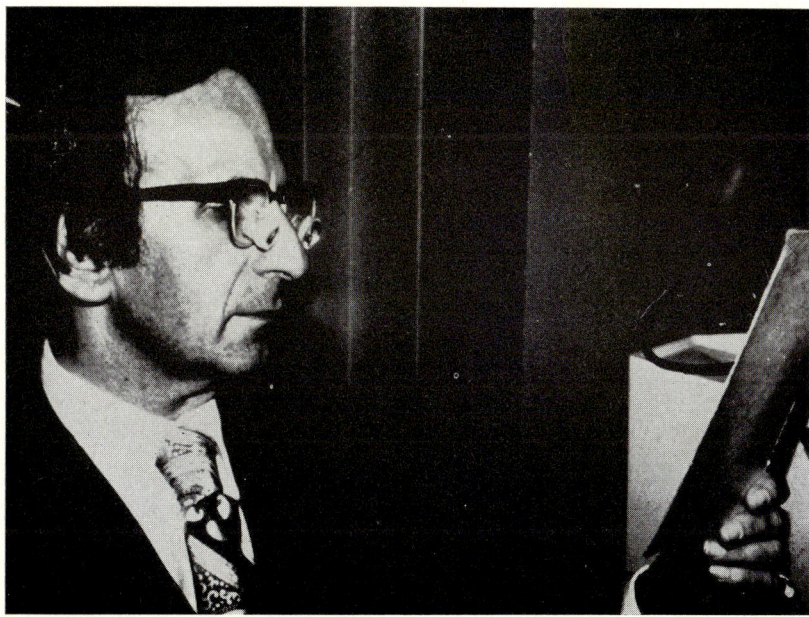

Figure XVII-6. 3.5x Telemicroscopic units used binocularly and set for a working distance of 16 in for his work as an attorney.

Case 5.
Patient: J.F., first seen in 1971 at age twenty-three.
Condition: uveitis, corneal dystrophy, OD, cataract, OS.
Distance Visual Acuity:
  Without correction: No LP, OD
                          5/125 OS.
  With correction: No LP, OD
                          5/77 OS.
                       with mydriatic.

This is the staff's favorite patient. He achieved so well in his college studies that he now has an administrative position at the same institution.

Aids Prescribed:
1. absorptive Photogray® corrective lenses.
2. Keeler 6x long-focus telemicroscopic spectacles which enabl patient to read 4-point type.
3. 2.2x Kollmorgen telescopic spectacles with +8 reading cap for desk work.
4. closed circuit television.
5. 6x15 hand held prism monocular telescope.

Case 6.
Patient: H.K., first seen in 1970 at age fifty-three.
Condition: OD, uveitis, aphakic, pupil updrawn.
                OS, endophthalmitis.
Distance Visual Acuity:
  without correction: 5/350, OD
                         No LP, OS.
  with correction: 10/100, OD
                         No LP, OS.

This housewife was discouraged about using her eyes after surgical intervention for removal of a cataract. Her aphakic spectacle enabled the patient to read newspaper size type using a closed circuit television. This instrument encouraged and provided the stimulus so necessary for vision rehabilitation. Several visits and an aphakic correction with a prism base-up allowed her to perform her household chores again. The prism was prescribed to align the visual axis with the updrawn pupil.

Aids Prescribed:
1. distance aphakic absorptive spectacles.

color—gray.
absorption—60 percent.
prism—4 △ base-up OD.
2. 8x microscopic spectacles which enabled patient to read 8-point type.

Case 7.
Patient: R.S., first seen in 1970 at age seventy-nine.
Condition: diabetic retinopathy, aphakia, OD.
           diabetic retinopathy, cataract, OS.
Distance Visual Acuity:
   without correction: 3/350 OD
                        10/150 OS.
   with correction: 2/400 OD
                        10/100 OS.

This is one of my favorite patients. She is a constant reminder that one can never place a limit on referrals for low vision evaluation, particularly in this case where a monocular aphakic correction could not be tolerated. A prescription for ordinary spectacles for the unoperated eye was recommended for constant wear, and her interest in sewing and reading was renewed with the use of low vision aids.

Aids Prescribed:
   1. distance absorptive spectacles.
      color—brown.
      absorption—55 percent.
   2. 5x hand magnifier for selection of groceries.
   3. 4x microscopic reading lens for 6-point type.
   4. 2.2x Kollmorgen telescopic spectacles for the theatre and television.
   5. 5 D neck magnifier for sewing and hooking rugs.

This patient now reads two books each week.

Absorptive Lenses and Prisms

In general, gray or brown shades of absorptive lenses are most commonly prescribed. However, in cases of peripheral loss as in glaucoma and retinitis pigmentosa, yellow lenses can be helpful. Since cones are the predominant visual receptor in the macular area and function most efficiently in bright illumination, their function is enhanced by this filter. Contrast is improved.

Occasionally prisms have special application in cases of peripheral

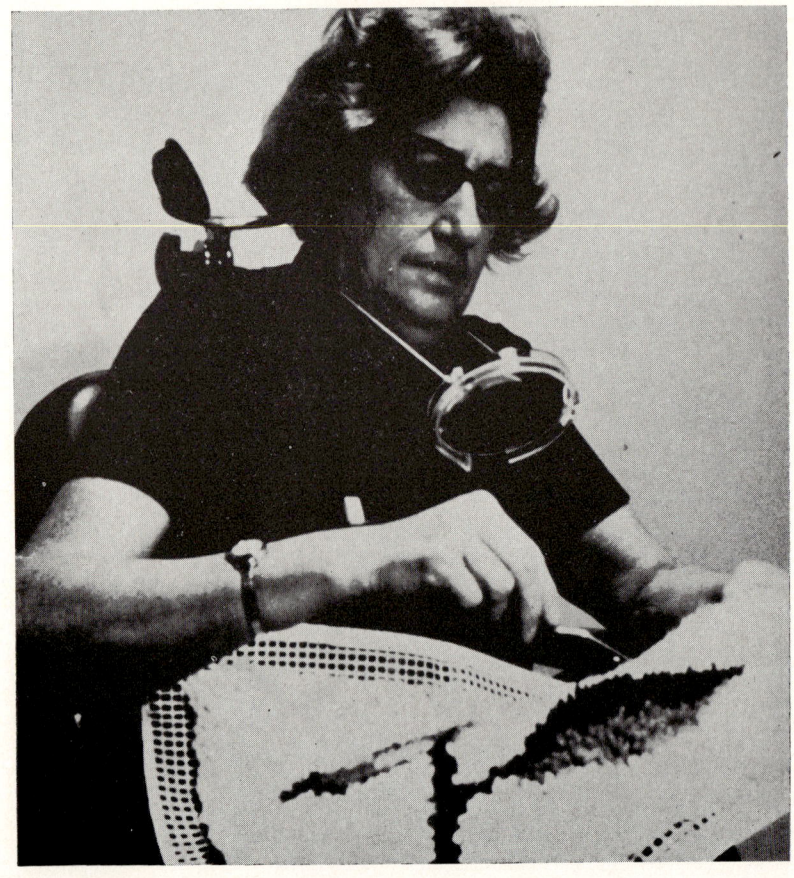

Figure XVII-7. A 5D neck magnifier allows this patient to continue her favorite pastime.

field loss. Base-*out* prisms are placed before each eye to utilize the temporal retina (nasal fields).

It has become a convention to prescribe base-in reading prisms in a half-eye frame, but an occasional patient may not be able to tolerate the half lens and will accept the same prism glass in a full frame.

Summary

Multiple visual aids are the modern concept of low vision precribing. Absorptive lenses and prisms are part of an ever increasing emphasis on sophisticated refinements in techniques.

· SECTION SIX ·
Vision Rehabilitation in the Geriatric Population

· CHAPTER XVIII ·

The Older Visually Limited Person: A Statistical Profile

Arlene R. Gordon

It is interesting to examine how a low vision service, set in the framework of a multiservice rehabilitation agency initially established for the blind, has contributed not only to a change in the focus and direction of the total agency but also to a greater awareness and understanding of the needs of a specific population.

A Low Vision Service, as with any rehabilitation service, needs to be constantly aware of the social, environmental, physical, and emotional factors prevailing in its patient population. This is true whether we are talking about the child, the vocationally bound adult, or the geriatric patient. In recognizing that demographic information is required to develop sound and valid programs, data-gathering and retrieval systems become an essential key in understanding the needs of a specific patient population. As a result, the NYAB, three years ago, began compiling for each year a statistical profile of its applicants for service. It would be helpful here to look at some of this information for the past year, 1972/73, in order to demonstrate more vividly not only the needs of the people but also the impact on program development.

Over one thousand individuals were registered for a variety of NYAB services. This does not include those who requested and obtained information and referral services. Fifty percent of the new cases were individuals of sixty-five years of age and over, a fact which points up the need for evaluation of services and programs for the steadily increasing geriatric group.

What degree of vision did this population have at the time they requested services? Of the 490 who were sixty-five years of age and over, only about twenty percent came with vision of less than

5/200, and of this number only twenty-four had light perception or less. This is a significant statistic which focuses attention on the change taking place in the older visually handicapped population. Almost half of the people seeking help are older people with some vision. Although a major function of an agency is still to meet the needs of people with severely reduced vision who may not be able to benefit from an aid, programs must be further refined to include the aging person with less than a total loss of vision. There must be not only awareness of the losses that accompany the loss of vision but also an awareness of the effects of the aging process so that, joined together with an understanding of the environment with which the individual must cope, the aging person can be helped to continue leading a meaningful life whether he is blind or partially sighted.

Moving on, then, to the purpose of this paper, one can state that the focus will be on the 389 individuals (eighty % of the applicants over sixty-five) who had significant residual vision and who were the applicants for and recipients of low vision services. The visual status at the time of the request was the following: of the group with over 5/200 vision, only 6 percent (twenty-three) had measurable vision between 5/200 and 10/200. Almost twenty-five percent (ninety-six) had vision between 10/200 and 20/200, and forty-eight percent (188) had an acuity of 20/200 or better or with restricted fields. Approximately twenty-one percent (eighty-two) had vision better than 20/200.

In summary, then, we are working with a population that is aging, that has lost some vision, a population that has had sight, a population that has visual memory and is still functioning on a visual basis. This means that agencies and rehabilitation services geared to the geriatric population have to have dual programs. There has to be a program for those who are totally blind or have minimal residual vision. But for the majority of people with usable sight who seek services, a different approach is called for. Our concern here is to describe the geriatric patient with reduced vision and to describe his social, environmental, and physical status in order to determine what supportive services will be necessary for a comprehensive program. This statistical profile will help us understand the patients, who, from all indications, should benefit from an aid and will assist us in offering guidance in their beginning adjustment as they organize their lives according to their individual capabilities and continue to be functioning members of their community.

In reviewing the characteristics of the total population over sixty-five (490), one-third (163) were living alone. Of the remaining two-thirds, 60 percent were living with families, foster families, and friends (only a small percent were individuals living with a spouse). The remaining 7 percent were in institutional or group-living arrangements. This means that the largest group of individuals, although with family and friends, were living for the most part in a dependent relationship in the family setting. Almost 50 percent (212) were widowed, with another 6.5 percent (sixty) persons single or divorced. This means that fifty-six percent of the individuals coming to the agency have suffered not only from loss of vision, but they have faced another loss in life, that of a spouse. They may also be suffering from other debilitating physical and/or emotional illnesses. These factors play a role in determining the counselling and supportive services that must be offered.

Looking next at the economic factors, we find that, of the group sixty-five years of age and over who were registered for services, 5 percent were employed, while only 8 percent were on welfare. The remaining 80 to 85 percent were living on social security income, savings, and pensions (a wide range of income, as there are many kinds of savings and many kinds of pensions). Our unrefined statistics in the area of finances indicate that a large proportion of these people were on marginal incomes.

We also know that thirty-five percent were not able to travel by themselves. The other sixty-five percent classified themselves as self-travelers. This brief sketch, broad in its statistical analysis, gives us a picture of the kind of population that comes to an agency in need of help in coping with reduced vision. We recognize that agencies have to overcome deep-seated attitudes which have prevailed in the community in the past and negative feelings about coming to a Low Vision Clinic or to an agency for the visually handicapped and blind.

It becomes evident that the person who takes the initiative in seeking the assistance of a low vision service, particularly one set in a rehabilitation agency for the visually handicapped or blind, is taking a major step in his own rehabilitation. It is the first step towards learning to control and master his own environment. Therefore, this population is more likely to have success with a low vision aid and, if and when the use of a low vision aid is not sufficient to restore visual functioning, is also more likely to be able to move on and benefit from other rehabilitation services.

It is essential that we evaluate the reasons for *failure* in those instances in which individual physical, social, and intellectual factors would all tend to support a prognosis of success.

The focus on the low vision geriatric patient, in an attempt to understand or gain a picture of that patient's capabilities and deficits, has led to reexamination of existing programs, a regrouping of available disciplines, and a refocusing of NYAB goals and objectives. Although we are dealing with the geriatric patient in this section, it should be remembered that the agency's understanding of the importance of using residual vision for all age groups has generally aided in the process of changing the thrust and direction of programs. When we see that a majority of individuals seeking agency services has some degree of residual vision, total rehabilitation has to take this into account.

With particular reference to the geriatric low vision population, we are aware that an agency-based program is not necessarily relevant to this group's needs. What is relevant is providing those backup services which will contribute towards the adjustment of the older patient with limited vision. This implies use as deemed appropriate of the social worker, the mobility specialist, and the rehabilitation teacher. In order to extend the services of the low vision clinic and to complete the rehabilitation process, it may be more important to assist the individual who, in the past, has participated in community programs by providing inservice training for the staffs of senior citizen centers, nursing homes, and other community resources. Public education for all disciplines which may have contact with the visually limited person contributes to the extension of more services to the visually handicapped.

Rehabilitation services to the older patient with reduced vision are measured in terms of individuals served. Educational services are measured in terms of improving the ability of professional and lay public to feel comfortable with and to be able to assist a blind and visually handicapped person.

The low vision clinic has brought an awareness of the importance of residual vision to this agency. Traditionally, before the more sophisticated approach of low vision workers, many people were classified as legally blind and were treated as blind when they possessed 20/200 vision. Present-day workers look at the potentialities of the visually handicapped person and the positive aspects of the person's ability to use whatever vision he has. By having as a focus the maximum use of residual vision, we realize that the majority of people within the legally blind classification do have a degree of vision and should be helped to use it. This in itself makes a tremendous difference in the way agencies and rehabilitation centers can revise and refocus their direction by never overlooking an important area, the attitudes of the community and the attitudes and fears people have because of the old myths that still prevail about blindness and loss of vision.

If we keep these attitudes in mind, we can understand that this is the reason why many people who have come to be known as the *hidden blind* are still reluctant to come for services.

If we improve public education by emphasizing the possibilities of the use of vision and by building better attitudes about the visually handicapped and the aging process and losses that may accompany it, then we stimulate new approaches towards services which are needed to ensure that the geriatric patient can live as a respected person in his community.

· CHAPTER XIX ·

Community Programs for the Visually Impaired Geriatric Patient

Leslie Fine

Introduction

THIS ARTICLE will attempt to describe some of the programs developed at our hospital for the elderly visually impaired patients and community residents. First, however, let me briefly describe the hospital. Coney Island Hospital in Southern Brooklyn is a municipal hospital of the City of New York that is affiliated with a voluntary hospital, Maimonides Medical Center. It services a large heterogeneous patient population which has one of the largest geriatric concentrations in the city, many of whom are poor and living marginal existences.

Demonstration Programs for the Elderly

In 1969 our hospital's department of psychiatry was awarded a three-year grant by the New York State Department of Mental Hygiene to fund a geriatric demonstration program whose broad-based mandate was to advocate, promote, provide, and evaluate services for the elderly in our hospital's catchment area. It was felt that our small staff's impact would be greatest if it gave high priority to the development of new services and programs which would be delivered by other agencies or in conjunction with our staff. It was within this framework that we were able to develop many new programs for the elderly, and, in particular for purposes of description for this article, specialized services for the elderly visually impaired patient.

Group Resocialization for the Blind

The first such service was a group resocialization program for the elderly blind which was established at our hospital jointly with Vacation and Community Services for the Blind, a nonprofit agency. This program currently services approximately forty-five elderly blind patients who are brought to the hospital once weekly for a four-hour program. Most of the patients were lonely, isolated, chronically depressed shut-ins. Many were in need of specialized medical, psychiatric social service, and rehabilitation, but they had not or could not avail themselves of such services. Some were known to the hospital clinics: many were not and were located via community outreach methods. The Vacation and Community Services provided a trained group worker, and our geriatric program provided two community workers, a social worker, an art therapist, and ten hospital volunteers to this group program. The services provided were therapeutic recreation and counseling services as well as assisted referrals to specialty services as the patients' needs were investigated and elaborated. The program thus served as the focus which brought the patients to the hospital and provided the staff to motivate and assist the patient in obtaining additional needed services. In this way it was felt that many of these patients could be maintained in the community as long as possible at an optimal level of functioning: they would otherwise, through neglect and deterioration, require hospitalization and/or institutionalization. This program did not materialize overnight: it presented many problems in interagency coordination, staff training and development, and hospital inertia. The greatest problem, one that had to be overcome in order to develop and maintain this program, was and is, however, the transportation system. Initially, Medicaid funding paid for transporting all the patients in the program to the hospital via four mini-buses which would pick up and return the patients to their homes. Then in 1971, when Medicaid funds were cut throughout New York City, this funding support was cut from our program and this service was in jeopardy. At this point the American Foundation for the Blind and subsequently some local Lions' Clubs were recruited to provide funding support for transportation for this program. The Lions' Clubs, in addition, were able to provide and deliver lunches for these patients during their group meeting. This was a welcome addition since many of these patients were not receiving proper nutrition at home, a euphemism to state that some of them were literally starving.

Vision-screening Clinic

A second program developed for the elderly was a series of demonstration vision-screening clinics which were developed and delivered by our geriatric staff and demonstrated how existing resources within the hospital and the community could be organized to deliver a new service. One of our geriatric community workers, because of her involvement with the hospital eye clinic and as part of her work with the blind resocialization group previously mentioned, learned that there were three community-oriented ophthalmology residents in the hospital who wanted to promote additional case material for their training and who had some spare time. Out of their interest it was possible for our staff to recruit and train a group of volunteers at a local senior center to administer visual acuity tests via Snellen charts and to complete a simple history and questionnaire devised by the eye residents. The staff also organized the publicity and coordinated the program so that these three residents were able to efficiently mass-screen three hundred elderly persons at a local senior center in a three-hour screening clinic. They found that approximately eighty persons had evidence of eye pathology which required further investigation and/or treatment. Of these eighty, fifty were referred to their local doctors, and thirty persons who had no private physician service available were referred back to the hospital eye clinic. There was, unfortunately, no follow-up to see how many referred patients actually followed up on their referral; and, if not, why not. This same mass-screening technique was repeated with smaller numbers of persons on three additional occasions at two different low-income housing projects for the elderly and one middle-income housing project for the elderly in our community. Although the same type of screening was done with two different income groups, the same type of yield was obtained as described above. Our department was besieged for some time after these clinics were held by local residents and by community groups asking if further screening would be done, and, if not, where they could obtain such services. This seemed to indicate the potential and the receptivity for future services on an ongoing basis to reach the large untapped numbers of elderly persons in our area.

Special Rehabilitative Services

A third cooperative program to provide services for the visually impaired in the hospital is currently being developed and will be started shortly. Our geriatric staff developed another cooperative program in which a social worker from the Industrial Home for the Blind, a nonprofit rehabilitation program for the blind, runs a group program at the hospital for recently blinded individuals, who are in need of special rehabilitative services but who are, for emotional reasons, unable and unwilling to accept a follow-up on such referrals. This group program will serve as a bridge enabling these individuals to overcome whatever resistances are operative in preventing such referrals from materializing. It is felt that such patients will more likely accept counseling help within a hospital setting rather than directly at the Industrial Home for the Blind.

Our geriatric staff has also been involved in curriculum development and the teaching of nurses aides and nurses within the hospital and within local nursing homes and homes for the aged on problems and care of the elderly, including care of the visually impaired and blind elderly. They have provided direct teaching of staff, have located educational materials including films, and have brought in experts in the field to talk to the trainees.

Our geriatric staff in conjunction with staff from our hospital's Community Medicine Department have also brought into the hospital continuing education programs for senior citizens. The teachers in this program are provided by Kingsborough Community College which is a branch of the City University of New York. The programs and curricula are chosen by the patients themselves via questionnaires. The applicants in the program are selected by nurses from the various clinics of the hospital and our own geriatric staff. Many of the visually impaired people known to us are also included in this mixed continuing education program. This program also serves as an additional resocialization outlet for intellectually intact people who otherwise would not go to the local community colleges. I might add that the reverse has also occurred: in addition to bringing educational programs into the hospital, our staff has also been asked to bring patients to educational programs outside of the hospital.

For example, the principal of a local school has asked if we could supply some visually impaired and blind individuals to teach children in his school about problems of the visually impaired as part of the school's community teaching program.

· CHAPTER XX ·

Care of the Elderly Low Vision Patient: Evaluation, Aids, Prognostic Factors

ALFRED A. ROSENBLOOM

Introduction

WHILE TODAY'S greater life expectancy is accompanied by a higher incidence of ocular and degenerative disorders, there is an increase in literacy among aging persons and an unwillingness by many of them to accept poor vision as a natural consequence of old age. Our nation's senior citizens are demanding that more attention be paid to their health care. Providing adequate vision care for the aging patient is a challenge to our professional skills and knowledge.

First, what essential understanding must we have about severely visually handicapped older patients if we are to gain a full appraisal of the total individual?

Second, do our examining techniques and procedures have to be modified in order to increase the reliability and validity of low vision testing?

Third, what prognostic factors should be considered during the visual rehabilitation of the aging patient?

Essential Understandings Concerning Severely Visually Handicapped Aged Patients

By definition, aging describes the physiological changes in a person's life from one point of time to another. Aging is a continuous process and, while developmental in nature, is highly individualized especially in the area of health problems.

One of the essentials in the field of geriatrics is that we should try to maintain the best degree of physical health and mental vigor for each person within the framework of aging. In this sense, rehabilitation is viewed as the restoration of an individual's ability to enjoy his life.

A second essential which the practitioner must realize is that the expectations for the social role of aged low vision patients should be similar to those applied to sighted persons, even though somewhat modified. The examiner should encourage the visually handicapped person to feel that it is possible to attain a reasonably happy and useful life, a degree of self-sufficiency, emotional independence, and satisfaction in social interactions with others. Too often our goals are physical in nature, and overlook these emotional, intellectual, and social aspects of life. The professional examiner must seek a rather complete understanding of the patient's visual needs and be constantly alert to the patient's personal goals.

Modification in Examination Techniques to Increase Reliability and Validity of Low Vision Findings

Every aspect of the low vision examination and aftercare carries important implications. The examination of the low vision patient is conducted in an observant manner. There are many clues which the examiner can recognize by the patient's entrance into the examining room. A preliminary assessment of the patient's ability to utilize functional vision can be made by noting if the patient must be led into the examining room or how he walks with his guide.

The initial contact with the professional examiner must provide time for the patient to discuss his visual difficulties and their meaning, if the visual condition is congenital or adventitious, and to ascertain how realistic are his goals. A good case history is vital to success in low vision care. Questions are directed to determine the patient's true low vision status, How is your general health? How long have you been visually handicapped? What is the medical diagnosis, treatment, and prognosis? Have you tried to use visual aids by yourself? Is reading an important activity to you? Do you use any magnifying lenses? Are there any special visual problems with which you would like us to help you?

Questions should be asked to establish the type of specific reading material the patient wishes to see and for what purpose. For the elderly patient, the most important qualities to establish from the history are his specific needs or desires, his ability to adapt to new situations, his motivation to learn new visual habits, and his understanding of the uses and limitations of the visual aid he will be using. If an elderly patient has lived with his family and has sighted persons around him, efforts may be directed to finding aids which will allow him to participate in normal family activities, e.g. TV, card playing, sewing, and games. However, if the patient lives alone, more attention may be focused on specific and necessary tasks such as reading mail, identifying labels on medicine, bottles or canned goods, and the activities that every person can enjoy such as TV, cards, and sewing.

At this point we try to establish the realistic levels of visual improvement which can be expected and to determine a preliminary judgment about the need for services with other members of the rehabilitation team. Thus for each individual there emerges a varying pattern of needs based on his individual situation and requiring the careful selection of the most appropriate low vision aid. If the elderly patient is capable of functioning in a realistic and effective manner, he will usually have needs and desires similar to those of more youthful patients. *Older people are not basically different* even though their problems, physical, psychological, and social in nature, may vary in degree and in kind.

Distance Testing

The diversity of low vision problems and individual needs requires great precision in the technical approach: the use of a sturdy trial frame and trial lenses; pinhole disc; stenopaic slit; Jackson cross cylinder ($\pm\ 0.50$ or $\pm\ 1.00$ D for astigmatic testing) distances of 10 feet or closer utilizing printed test cards. Appropriate illumination controls are essential items of examining equipment and increase the sensitivity and accuracy of a patient's responses.

The testing environment must be carefully structured so that the patient can achieve with ease the recognition of at least one line of letters or numbers. It is not uncommon with elderly patients to determine a subjective refraction which sometimes differs significantly from the patient's habitually worn correction. A carefully determined subjective examination frequently provides improved mobility and travel vision.

High refractive corrections, be they aphakic or highly myopic in power, have effective power characteristics related to their base curve, center thickness, and vertex distance. The Halberg clips which are attached to the habitual correction provide an effective approach to over-refraction. The spherocylindrical correction determined in conjunction with the spectacle correction can then be accurately determined by placing both the habitual and the newly determined lens powers in the lensometer which provides the practitioner with the resultant correction. Final refinement of the distance correction with a low power afocal telescopic lens provides not only a measurable and qualitative improvement in visual acuity but also serves as a means for verifying with greater accuracy the tentative distance correction.

Clinical results with elderly patients have emphasized the need for the practitioner to be constantly aware that, no matter how limited a patient's vision may be, vision and its limitations are what he lives and functions with. Therefore, if his vision can be improved even slightly, the patient's whole perspective and outlook improve and the scope of his rehabilitation is broadened.

Near Testing

Near testing is carried out at the focal point of the lens or lens combination, disregarding accommodation. Following the determination of the magnification power needed on a standardized test card, realistic reading matter is then substituted for the reading card in the form of a newspaper, book, or magazine.

Lighting is carefully determined in relation to level of intensity and visual need. The quality of illumination: diffuseness characteristic, background and contrast, presence of glare, is another essential consideration.

Having decided that a patient can benefit from a low vision aid, the practitioner must be certain that the patient is properly trained in its use. Inherent limitations in the visual aids themselves require adaptation to such factors as working distance, field of vision, and spatial distortions. New motor patterns of coordination involving head, hand, and eye must be learned. For elderly patients, this frequently is a more difficult task with a spectacle type of aid and often dictates the prescription of simpler, less complex visual aids: for example, a fixed focus or focusable hand or stand magnifier.

Since low vision prescription is primarily task and interest oriented, the use of a single aid to fulfill multiple needs is seldom possible. For this reason, multiple aids are frequently used to provide variations in magnification, viewing distance, size of field, and flexibility in use. The dispensing of a final prescription should be postponed until the patient has demonstrated the ability to read. He should be familiar with the appearance of the visual aid, be able to perform desired, useful tasks, and demonstrate proficiency in its use.

The dispensing of a low vision aid does not necessarily conclude the practitioner's responsibility. Does the patient appear to need other services? He may need orientation and mobility instruction for independent travel. He may also need psychological evaluation, financial assistance, or home teaching including talking book services. The aging person frequently experiences a markedly different role, from a parent-provider to a less authoritarian, more dependent relationship. Marked visual impairment often intensifies feelings of dependency, inadequacy, and perhaps hostility. The examiner must recognize this changing role and refer the patient to social service workers who can give both the individual and his family counseling and guidance towards a more positive attitude, one of understanding, acceptance, and an awareness of altered interpersonal relationships.

It is imperative that the examiner or his staff know the variety of services available and the sources for obtaining them. For example, The American Foundation for the Blind publishes a manual entitled *Directory of Agencies Serving the Visually Handicapped in the U. S.* which lists, by state, the types of services available and the agencies, both public and private, which provide these services.

Prognostic Factors in the Rehabilitation of Aging Patients

A group of 276 low vision patients drawn at random from two thousand patients who had been examined and prescribed low vision aids in the Low Vision Clinic of the Chicago Lighthouse for the

Blind, received follow-up care within six months to one year after the date of the original examination and dispensing of the low vision aid. The purpose of the examination was to evaluate the patient's success in maintaining the gains in visual efficiency which were characteristic of the original examinaton.

The patients ranged in age from sixty to eighty-nine years; eighty percent were between the ages of sixty and seventy-nine, while twenty percent were eighty years of age or older. This follow-up study revealed that approximately seventy-six percent of the patients continued to use the low vision aid and reported moderate to highly successful results. In 24 percent of the cases, the patients had discontinued the use of the low vision aid. The group classified as highly successful comprised 44 percent of the patients. These were individuals who wore the low vision aid regularly, performed a variety of visual tasks from day to day, and were highly enthusiastic and happy with the results. The patients judged moderately successful comprised 32 percent of the sample. These individuals did not wear their aid constantly but reported using them regularly for their intended purposes.

Two groups of patients were identified among the 24 percent considered to be unsuccessful. A small group of 9 percent may have been able to continue using their low vision aids; however, senile changes, poor health, or a loss in vision had seriously limited their use of and enthusiasm for the visual aid. The remaining 15 percent of the patients seldom wore the aid or expressed any interest in returning for reexamination. It is interesting to note that among the thirty patients over eighty years of age, 60 percent benefited from their low vision aids.

How do we cope with failure? In patients who present the potential for success but reject the low vision aid, we most often observe individuals who have recently lost their vision and who perhaps have not totally accepted their visual loss.

In evaluating the clinical results of this older group, we also noted in some cases that their needs, adaptive capabilities, interests, and physical problems produced limitations which were distinct from their vision problems. In such cases the social worker, psychologist, or psychiatrist is an important figure in the rehabilitation process.

Group therapy or individual counseling may help the patient achieve an understanding and an acceptance of his visual loss and other limitations.

It is also interesting to note that certain low vision aids are used more successfully than others. Within the successful outcome group, approximately two thirds of the patients were prescribed either a microscopic lens ranging in power from 3x to 15x or a high plus reading addition ranging in power from +4.00 D to +14.00 D. The near vision of over 80 percent of these patients was improved to the point at which magazine and newsprint could be read. Approximately 12 percent of the aids prescribed involved the use of fixed or focusable stand magnifiers. Selection of this aid was often dictated by senile changes or occupational preference and by the inabilities to adapt successfully to precise fixation-coordination of a headborne aid or to the uses of an interim or auxiliary correction. Telescopic units, often of the ready-made type, were prescribed successfully in 10 percent of the cases.

There is no area of professional practice that offers greater possibility for humanitarian service. Low vision care provides the opportunity for widening the scope of professional activity and the possibility for making full, creative use of the techniques and aids already developed. The low vision team can be rightfully proud of its technological and clinical achievements. Here then is the challenge for the professional examiner, his trained assistant, and his colleagues in related disciplines to give more low vision patients the opportunity to rediscover their vision.

Suggested Reading List

Brazelton, Frank A., Stamper, Bruce, and Stern, Victor: Vocational rehabilitation of the partially sighted. *Am J Optom*, 47(8): 612-18, 1970.

Hirsch, M. J., and Wick, R. E.: *Vision of the Aging Patient*. Philadelphia, Chilton, 1960. Chapter 10: Partial Vision and Optical Aids, Chapter 15: Social and Vocational rehabilitation of the blind and partially sighted older patient.

Mehr, Edwin B., and Mehr, Helen: Psychological factors in working with partially sighted persons. *Journal of the American Optometric Association, 40(8)* : 842-46, 1969.

Mehr, Helen M., Mehr, Edwin B., and Ault, Carroll: Psychological aspects of low vision rehabilitation. *Am J Optom, 47(8)* : 605-12, 1970.

Rosenberg, Robert: Training in low vision practice. *Journal of the American Optometric Association, 39(1):57-60, 1968.*

Rosenbloom, Alfred A.: Subnormal vision problems of the aging patient. *Optometric Weekly, 51(46)* :2403-09, 1960.

Rosenbloom, Alfred A.: Prognostic factors in the visual rehabilitation of aging patients. *The New Outlook for the Blind, 68(3)* : 124-27, 1974.

Shorr, Robert H., Gaynes, Ernest M., and Honeyman, Max M.: System of rehabilitation of partially sighted patients. *Am J Optom, 49(4)* : 368-71, 1972.

Zettle, John, Jr.: The care of low vision. *Am J Optom, 41(3)* : 142-49, 1964.

· SECTION SEVEN ·
Driving with Telescopes

Alan H. Barnert

Introduction

Driving with special optical aids means driving with telescopes, and that entails accepting the fact that there is more than one approach to the role that vision plays in safe driving. Opinions in the following papers vary from supportive to negative. There is obviously a need to examine standards and attitudes with a fresh approach and to try to organize a fair set of standards which will not be prejudicial against the visually limited person, the driving public or the pedestrian.

The situation is as follows. Cars have to be driven by people; even a sophisticated computer cannot drive a car. All of the states have physical requirements for licensing people to drive, and all have visual requirements although these vary from state to state. Obviously it takes a certain amount of vision to drive a car. Since our society is built around the motorcar, it is extremely important that each individual be allowed to drive if he can do so without danger to himself or to others. It is important in work and in living in general, as well as in recreation and play. What happens to the borderline case in which vision is slightly reduced and driving is essential? It evolves that there is a method involving telescopes that enables borderline people to pass the standards and to drive while wearing these telescopes. But since these devices have limitations which may not have been foreseen or permitted when the standards were set up, the questions are, Should such people be licensed to drive cars? Should people be allowed to drive wearing telescopes if they cannot pass the requirements without them? And of course there are a number of subsidiary questions, What standards should be set? Should there be any restrictions on driving such as speed, night driving, special equipment? How is the selection, training, and testing of such persons done?

These questions will be treated in the following chapters.

· CHAPTER XXI ·

The Rationale for Licensure: Criteria and Training

Julian D. Newman

In major metropolitan areas, public transportation is available. In most smaller communities this is usually not the case, yet the population of all communities needs mobility for economic and social intercourse. This population includes the partially sighted who lack the necessary mobility because of inability to obtain a motor vehicle license.

The rationale for investigating some form of legal licensure for some of the partially sighted is whether it is better to grant a license or to adhere to restrictive laws which waste human potential and increase the welfare rolls.

Frequently persons with low vision drive without benefit of licenses, and jeopardize the economic security of their families. In fact, it has been the experience of this writer that the greatest majority of low vision population with acuities of 20/200 or better have had some driving experience without benefit of licensure. There is no standardization of static visual acuity requirements in the United States. Some states require best corrected vision of 20/40, some 20/70. According to Edward Wade, the director of the Drivers License Division in North Carolina, people can be licensed with vision as low as 20/100 with the restrictions of no night driving and maximum speed of 45 miles per hour (mph). Although the visual standards of North Carolina are lower than the other forty-nine states, the accident rate in the state is no higher than average for the United States.

A proposed criterion for licensing low vision drivers is more or less an acceptance of the acuity standards of North Carolina. A licensing candidate with a best corrected visual acuity of 20/100 in each eye correctable to 20/40 when using a telescopic lens and a 140° peripheral field can be considered.

Albert Burg[1] of the University of California at Los Angeles and Robert Henderson of the Systems Development Corporation are presently doing research in the area by defining the relationship between certain aspects of vision and driving performance. Their research has shown that there is a high correlation between reduced static visual acuity and poor driving performance in the age group over fifty-five and that in the age groups below fifty-five there is low correlation between static visual acuity and driving performance.

The goal of the Burg-Henderson research is to establish new visual criteria for applicants for driver's licensing and to develop instruments to measure these criteria.

Low Vision License Candidates

Clinically the writer has found that approximately 3 percent of his low vision patients meet his criteria for licensure. These criteria are:

1. Applicant must need a license for employment or will suffer extreme hardship.
2. Applicant has undergone a rigorous and extensive driver's training program before being licensed.
3. Applicant must wear the Bioptic when driving; Bioptic preferably should be a wide-angle type of no more than 3.0x in power; and the exterior of the lens should be painted black to reduce the halo effect in the telescope.
4. Best corrected acuity through the Bioptic portion must be 20/40 in each eye.
5. Vehicle must have side view mirrors.
6. No night driving.
7. Peripheral fields of 140° laterally.
8. License is for one year only with an annual reexamination.

A possible method of adapting and training the low vision licensing candidate would be as follows.

> The candidate must first wear the Bioptic lens system for thirty days and learn the technique of spotting objects through the telescopic portion.

Then the patient must receive a temporary learner's permit allowing him to drive in off-street areas such as those used in driver's education training courses. After showing proficiency, the candidate must receive a regular learner's permit for on-street driving for ninety days and finally submit himself to an extensive road test. Once he has passed, the candidate can receive the special one-year license.

The Bioptic consists of a carrier lens with patient's distance correction and a telescope mounted high in the carrier with the distance correction also included in the telescope. The telescope is used merely for spotting signs and objects that are not clear. The driver is usually looking through the nontelescopic portion when driving which gives him the full, unobstructed field in the periphery.

Safety Record of Low Vision Drivers

The State of Massachusetts with 128 low vision drivers has had the greatest experience in licensure. In the period from June 1, 1967 to May 1, 1973, 341 man-years of driving were logged by these low vision drivers. During that time these drivers were involved in five accidents (in only one accident was the low vision driver found to be at fault), or one accident per 68.2 man-years of driving. The rate of accidents among the normally sighted population in Massachusetts was one accident per 17.6 man-years of driving. Thus the low vision driving population's safety record was four times better than that of normally sighted population.[2]

The real and ever present danger of a low vision driver being involved in a fatal accident (whether charged or not charged in the accident) creates a great moral responsibility for the practitioner who recommended licensure and has legal ramifications for the state agency issuing the licenses. According to Dr. Carter Tallman, a fatality has been reported recently involving a low vision driver in the State of Massachusetts; at this time, cause and responsibility have not been determined. Much more research must be done before a definitive answer can be given. However, the driving privilege which ensures the right to economic freedom should not be automatically granted or denied until further research is done in this area and experiences of practitioners are analyzed and correlated.

REFERENCES

1. Burg, A.: Vision and driving: a report on research. *Human Factors,* *13(1)*: 79-87, 1971.
2. Korb, D.: Preparing the visually handicapped person for motor vehicle operation. *Am J Optom,* *47*(8), 1970.

CHAPTER XXII

A Positive Approach to Driving With Telescopic Glasses

CARTER B. TALLMAN

Introduction

WITH NINETY-ONE million licensed drivers in the United States and an ever increasing dependence on the automobile for travel, there is an obvious interest in understanding what visual parameters are related to safe driving or a low crash record. At the present time, visual requirements for obtaining a driver's license vary from state to state. A personal survey revealed varying requirements for visual acuity in the best eye for a Class 3 license (operating a private automobile not for hire) in various states (See Table XXII-I).

TABLE XXII-I
VISUAL ACUITY REQUIREMENTS BY STATES

Visual Acuity	Number of States
20/20	1
20/30	7
20/40	36
20/50	3
20/60	1
20/70	1
20/100	1

Restricted licenses for daylight driving only are commonly allowed for persons with visual acuities up to 20/70 in many of these states. Other parameters occasionally tested included color vision and visual field.

Telescopes for driving are allowed in twenty-three states.

Suggested Vision Standards for Licensure

The American Medical Association committee on special aspects of automotive safety[1] set forth the following suggested standards of vision for operators with a Class 3 license.

Visual Acuity: 20/40. Spectacle correction of 10 diopters or more in the better eye is disqualifying unless horizontal field of 180° can be demonstrated.

Field of Vision: with a 6/1000 white target, a 30° field to each side of fixation with both eyes open is required or with a 2/330 white target a total field of 140° with both eyes open is required.

Color Vision: test of color discrimination not required.

Stereopsis: not required.

Associated Ocular Pathology: certain diseased states of the eye which cause difficulty with night vision are mentioned here. These include opacities and scars of the media, fixed or irregular pupils, pigmentary degenerations of the retina, papilledema, and tumors of the eye.

Arthur Keeney, M.D.,[2] a member of the committee, feels that the presence of most of these diseases indicates the need for a restricted daylight license.

Heterophoria: not disqualifying unless driver must close one eye to avoid diplopia.

Although these standards may appear prudent, it is important to realize that there is *very little data* to back up these suggestions. Arthur Keeney[3] states that there is no statistical evidence to justify 20/40 as a visual requirement for driving. However, Keeney[4] feels that 20/40 should be a requirement and feels that one argument for required 20/40 visual acuity is the new highway signs which are supposedly engineered to be seen easily by a person with 20/40 vision driving at the posted speed limit. A study by the Indiana State Police shows that persons with less vision have the best driving record. Massachusetts lost a golden opportunity to evaluate the crash record of persons with a visual acuity between 20/50 and 20/70 when their stiffer visual requirement of 20/40 came into effect. The ophthalmic community requested the Registry of Motor Vehicles to compare the crash records of those people who lost their licenses during the previous year with that group which was allowed to keep their license. Unfortunately, this study was never undertaken. Burg[5,6] correlated a reduced dynamic visual acuity with increased crash experience.

Unfortunately, this is not a basic clinical tool at the present time. It is obvious that more studies must be done before rational standards can be set.

The Bioptic System for Licensure

A telescopic system which is applicable for automobile driving is the Bioptic system reported by Feinbloom in 1958.[7] It consists of the spectacle lens correction and a compact telescopic system mounted through the top of the spectacle correction. The patient's own correction can be mounted on the back of the telescope. With the wearer's head in the primary position, the visual axis passes through the spectacle correction. When the head is slightly lowered, the visual axis passes through the telescopic system. Either the spectacle lens correction or the telescopic correction may be selected at any time for best vision with minimal changes in head position. The field of vision is about 8° while looking through the telescope for a 3x correction.

The Bioptic telescopic system is used in the following manner while driving an automobile. With this system the patient does 99 percent of his driving using his normal glasses correction and reduced visual acuity. The telescopic portion is used for only one-to two-second intervals for spotting and reading signs. Thus, when prescribing this system one makes the basic assumption that a person is able to drive safely with the visual acuity that is less than the minimum requirement of his or her state.

Korb[8] in 1970 reported the results from the twenty-six persons who received driver's licenses in the state of Massachusetts using the Bioptic telescopic system. Massachusetts requires a visual acuity of 20/40 through standard correction or telescopic lenses in order to receive a license. There are presently about 160 licensed drivers in Massachusetts wearing telescopic glasses. There have been three accidents with only one possibly due to driver error.

In an effort to see how effective the Bioptic system is for my patients, I have followed ten patients from one to twelve months. All but one of these patients have used the glasses and continued to drive. The patient who discontinued driving is a seventy-year-old gentleman with macular degeneration and an aphakic correction corrected by contact lenses and a Bioptic telescopic system worn over these. Although he passed the driver's test including a two hour driving test in downtown Boston by wearing the glasses, he felt that he was not a safe driver and discontinued driving. One nineteen-year-old boy with 20/200 vision had a minor unreported accident. This was due to an error in judgment and not related to his visual problem. He went around a rotary in the wrong direction as a lark and was involved in a minor fender-bender accident. This is a good example that perhaps judgment is far more important than vision when it comes to safe driving. Another person with 20/70 vision states that she does not need the glasses when driving in familiar areas and does not use the glasses except for driving in areas in which the reading of street signs becomes important. Interestingly, she obtained her license with the telescopic lenses; but her picture was not taken with the telescopic lenses, and it was not recorded on her driver's license.

My group of drivers drove anywhere from twenty to two hundred miles on an average per week. In general, on super highways they drove at the speed limit. In town they tended to drive at the speed limit or slightly less. Most felt that the easiest driving was on the highway. They felt that highway signs, in general, were constructed so that they had plenty of time to see the sign and read it even without the telescopic lenses. However, the telescopic lenses do allow them to see the signs sooner and therefore have an even greater reaction time. In-town driving, the changing back and forth from telescopic vision to natural vision, was sometimes difficult because of the closeness of traffic.

The telescopic lens portion is used for reading street signs, occasionally seeing street lights especially when they are in the sun, identifying policemen's hand signals, checking intersections at a distance, and looking ahead on a highway. They are *not used continuously* while driving, nor are they used for seeing cars or pedestrians. Road signs, such as STOP and SLOW, are usually seen without telescopic glasses.

When asked to compare the use of telescopic glasses to another driving aid (use of the sideview mirror), all stated that with practice the telescopic lenses take the same or less time than does the use of the sideview mirror. This is very significant since it indicates how little time is necessary to spot objects adequately through the telescopes. Both tasks become routine, and both involve momentarily averting the eyes from the road directly ahead.

The concensus is that the telescopic glasses allow the drivers to be safer with greater reaction time than if they were not wearing the glasses at all.

All drivers felt reasonably comfortable driving with their reduced visual acuity; and, if given a license without telescopic lenses, they would probably do some driving. However, all the drivers felt that the telescopic lenses are a distinct aid in driving. The drivers in this study generally did not drive at night, although circumstances might require them to drive at that time. I do not think that they should receive a restricted daytime license.

My present criteria for prescribing telescopic glasses are as follows.
1. Visual acuity of 20/50 to 20/200.
2. Field of vision of 140° with both eyes open.
3. An apparently reliable individual with a definite need to drive.
4. No obvious other physical handicaps such as coordination problems.

My present procedure for prescribing telescopic glasses for driving is as follows.
1. Distance glasses fit with the Bioptic 2.2x, 3.0x, or 4.0x telescope at the top of the lens set at the distance P.D..
2. A 2.2x or 3.0x telescope is used if this will give 20/40 acuity easily. Otherwise a 4.0x telescope is used.
3. The patient practices with the glasses for three months at home and as a passenger in an automobile.
4. The patient returns after three months for a reevaluation examination. This examination determines if the patient has 20/40 acuity with the telescopes and if he is able to make rapid adjustments between the telescopic and the standard lens portion of his glasses.
5. A letter is then sent with the patient to the Registry of Motor Vehicles requesting an exam for licensure.

6. In Massachusetts, upon passing the visual requirements with his telescopic lenses, the patient receives an unrestricted license, showing his picture with the telescopic glasses.

Summary

1. Ten persons with visual acuities ranging from 20/60 to 20/200 who received telescopic glasses for driving are presented.
2. Nine out of ten are successful drivers. One retired voluntarily.
3. Driving skills and good judgment are probably more important than 20/40 visual acuity.
4. All persons with vision of 20/60 or less who are going to drive should be considered candidates for telescopic glasses.
5. The Bioptic telescopic system seems a reasonable and prudent method of enabling persons with less than *legal* vision to drive a car.
6. More conclusive studies are needed to determine what physical characteristics can be reasonably tested and what characteristics are necessary for safe driving.
7. We should make every effort to maintain the visually handicapped on the road as long as this seems in the best interests of our patients and society at large. The right to drive is too important a privilege to remove without just cause.

REFERENCES

1. Committee on Medical Aspects of Automotive Safety: Visual factors in automobile driving and provisional standards. *Arch Ophthalmol, 81*: 865-87, 1969.
2. Keeney, A.: Relationship of ocular pathology and driving impairment. *Trans Pac Acad Ophthalmol Otolaryngol, 21*: 22-27, 1968.
3. Keeney, A.: Ophthalmology in driving. *Trans Pac Coast Otoophthalmol Soc, 51*: 167-78, 1967.
4. Personal communication, 1973.
5. Burg, A.: Vision and driving: a report on research. *Human Factors, 13(1)*: 79-87, 1971.
6. Burg, A.: The relationship between vision test scores and driving records. *General Findings,* report number 67-24, June, 1967.
7. Feinbloom, W.: The bioptic telescopic system. Paper read before the Section on Contact Lenses and Subnormal Vision, December, 1958, American Academy of Optometry.
8. Korb, D.: Preparing the Visually Handicapped Person for Motor Vehicle Operation. *Am J Optom, 47(8)*: 619-28, 1970.

· CHAPTER XXIII ·

Experience of A Low Vision Patient Driving With a Bioptic Telescope

Dennis K. Kelleher

Licensure Prerequisites

I. Before a candidate can be considered for driving with the Bioptic telescope, we suggest the following prerequisites compiled from the criteria used by Korb[1] in Massachusetts and Kelleher[2] in California. The most important of the criteria in our opinion is the visual fields requirement.
   A. Full visual fields of at least 110° with no large scotomas. (A bowl perimeter is the method of choice in Massachusetts and California for determining this.)
   B. A visual condition which is stable and preferably one which is congenital or of long duration.
   C. Normal color perception.
   D. Normal eye motility.
   E. Adequate central visual acuity to meet minimum requirements as prescribed by the state licensing law with the aid of the Bioptic.
   F. A sense of high moral responsibility. (Although this is somewhat intangible and difficult to evaluate, it was thought desirable to select individuals who would voluntarily restrict themselves from driving in conditions dangerous to themselves and others. Although their license may not restrict them, it was hoped that low vision drivers would not attempt to drive directly into the sun on a congested freeway or on icy roads at night.)
   G. A highly motivated and intelligent individual who has a need to drive for employment or for independence. (Since one actually *sees* with his brain, it follows that an intelligent per-

sons's brain will learn to interpret potential dangers more often and more rapidly.)

Fitting the Bioptic

II. Important subjective considerations in fitting the Bioptic are the following.
 A. Pupillary distance, is important if there is a bilateral prescription of the Bioptic unit and binocularity is to be attempted. In our opinion precise collimation of the optical axes of the telescopic systems is difficult if not impossible for most low vision patients.[1,2]

 If low vision patients are monocular, obviously only one telescopic unit need be prescribed. If the patient alternates or suppresses one eye, there may be several advantages to a binocular prescription. For example, the author uses a +2.00 D cap over his right telescope for reading the instrument panel, the odometer, fuel gauge, and temperature gauge. (The speedometer can be seen through the *carrier* lens.) The left telescope is used in the usual way for driving.

 If the low vision patient had normal binocular vision before his vision loss, he may need a binocular fitting to avoid diplopia especially if the acuity is nearly the same in each eye.
 B. The angle of the Bioptic is important to some patients. When the Bioptic is mounted normally at the lab, it is set at about a 10° superior angle. By lowering this angle to between 5° and 0° the patient increases the optical jump between telescopic and regular field so that moving an object of regard from one field to another can be done with a minimum of head movement and maximum of eye movement. Since the eye moves approximately ten times faster than the head, the time advantage when driving becomes self-evident. Another alternative to changing the placement angle of the Bioptic unit in the carrier is to introduce appropriate amounts of prism base-down over the objective.
 C. Vertex distance should be minimized to yield the largest possible field through the telescope.
 D. The effect upon nystagmus if present should also be con-

sidered, e.g. Bioptics are always positioned in the superior portion of the carrier lens for driving. If the nystagmus frequency and/or amplitude increases upon a superior angle of gaze, it should be noted that this might adversely affect visual efficiency.

E. Horizontal placement of the Bioptic unit is another critical consideration. By moving the Bioptic as little as 1 or 2 mm laterally or nasally, acuity might sharply drop off especially when strabismus is present.

Driving Problems Using the Bioptic

III. Some of the problems cited by Korb[1] and others in using the Bioptic for driving are discussed.

A. Head, neck, and eye coordination become second nature for the low vision patient using the Bioptic telescope to drive. The author has several Bioptics, some with prism and some without; yet, he can readily alternate, and after one or two attempts at aligning things in the small magnified field, the problem of alignment and amount of movement of the head, eyes, and neck is quickly adjusted.

B. Telescopic parallax and ring scotomas are a problem but not a significant one. One soon learns to judge distance through the telescope by merely rapidly fixating through the magnified and unmagnified portions of the lens system. In this way it it possible to judge depth monocularly. This can also be achieved by maintaining a reference point in the peripheral field while fixating through the Bioptic telescope. Though it may sound somewhat dubious to the non-low vision individual, the ring scotoma can be ignored in most situations. The eye can alternate fixation very rapidly, and the head can also change direction and move the blocked-out area of the field so that each successive picture received by the brain is different. The closest analogous situation would be that of a normally sighted person who has only one eye and who is never disturbed by his physiological blind spot.

C. Mirrors and vibrations are another consideration, but here again the low vision patient can learn to compensate adequately for them.

D. Illumination for some drivers with low vision is a definite problem. There are numerous eye shades, visors, and other means to minimize this problem.

I do not mean to imply by the above remarks that I do not feel that these things present any problem. Rather, these problems are possibly not fully understood by those not having low vision, and, consequently, their magnitude might be somewhat overestimated. These are all problems which deserve special considerations, but they can all be compensated for by the resourceful low vision patient.

Nonoptical Considerations

IV. Other considerations of a nonoptical nature might include one or more of the following.
  A. Illumination is generally an important factor for the motor vehicle operator who has low vision. Light direction and intensities fluctuate quite frequently. A dark-colored car with a nonreflective hood and dark dashboard area and car interior might be suggested for the photophobic driver. Other suggestions include tinted windshield and/or tinted glass all around the vehicle, broad-brimmed hat, and movable and oversized sunvisors in the car. The eye specialist might also prescribe a black housing on the Bioptic instead of clear plastic to minimize side light interference. The carrier and Bioptic might be tinted a light #1 pink or gray for the light sensitive driver.
  C. A small compact or subcompact car is suggested since it would be more maneuverable and give the low vision driver a greater advantage in depth and width perception. A vehicle with a sloping hood or one in which the driver sits in a low position in relation to the hood would not be recommended because of the lack of a reference point and the invisibility of a large ground area directly in front of the hood.
  D. A standard transmission is not essential but might be advisable since it allows the driver more control over speed and braking at low speed when the car is in lower gear. This also offers the low vision driver better control in slow, city street driving, driving on mountain curves and hills, and driving under such adverse conditions as snow, rain, or fog when reduced speed

enables the use of a lower gear and results in better control of the vehicle.

Driving Recommendations

V. Advice relative to driving a motor vehicle with low vision is as follows.
- A. Keep eyes constantly moving to scan the everchanging road situation.
- B. Do not look down over the front fender but as far ahead as possible to get a larger perspective.
- C. If the first two suggestions are explicitly followed you will automatically be doing the third suggestion. Be sure you are getting the whole picture of what is going on.
- D. Be sure the other drivers see you. If in doubt, blink your lights or blow your horn.
- E. If all else fails, leave yourself an escape. Do not tailgate.
- F. Keep your vehicle in good mechanical working order.
- G. Keep the mirrors and the windshields both back and front clean and dust free inside and out to maximize visibility.
- H. Never drive with any distractions which inhibit sensory input. A blasting radio which blocks auditory cues to the low vision driver is dangerous since the person with impaired vision often compensates for this loss by using auditory means more effectively.
- I. Never drive while under the influence of alcohol or any medications which impair reaction time.

A through E above are suggestions for good defensive driving from the Institute of Driver Behavior. Letters G through I above were compiled by Kelleher[2] in California and Korb[1] in Massachusetts on a low vision driver population of over 135. None of the sample would operate a motor vehicle even after one drink. Over one hundred of the sample reported that they would not operate a vehicle with dirty windshields or mirrors or if there was a distraction, especially an auditory one.

Training Procedures

VI. Training procedures employed are the following.

It was felt by the author and others [1,2] that full proficiency in the use of the Bioptic telescope (especially for driving which is a highly visually sophisticated task) requires use of the device for at least thirty hours. This training was usually from one to two hours daily for a minimum of one month. Some individuals needed more time to adjust to the Bioptic than others. In order to demonstrate proficiency, driving candidates instructed by the author in California had to ride in a car as a passenger and announce potential hazards and situations requiring definitive action as if the patient were driving. Upon passing this initial evaluation in using the Bioptic, the individual was permitted to apply to the Division of Motor Vehicles to take the state eye exam for a learner's permit.

To lead up to this efficient use of the Bioptic, four sequential steps were taken.

1. The subject was instructed to locate stationary objects by aligning the object of regard directly below the Bioptic field and then moving the eye and head slightly to view the object through the Bioptic.
2. Each subject was then taught to track moving objects in much the same way. Subjects would locate the object in their large field, anticipate its movement, and move the eye and head in a coordinated fashion (possibly diagonally or obliquely) to view the object through the Bioptic. When this became a quick yet smooth motion, almost instinctive on the part of the individuals, the next level of training was started.
3. Activities to promote visual memory were introduced. This was an effort to train the brain to be selective while being bombarded by many stimuli. At the same time, retention was stressed. The duration of exposure to the stimuli was constantly diminished to intervals of not more than one second in order to simulate short fixation times while driving.
4. Finally, levels of illumination were changed while the subject attempted to track and recognize and retain visual information. Activities which had previously been conducted under constant illumination indoors were now attempted outside at different angles to the sun and at different times of day.

Suitable targets for the above training procedures included flashcards, pictures, numbers, different-shaped signs of specific colors e.g., a yellow diamond-shaped sign with two fairly long words was not usually recognized on first exposure because the subject attempted to read it. On later exposures it was recognized as a "dangerous intersection" because of the word length, type of sign, and context of the situation.

Visual recognition of the instrument panel was trained in much the same way. As one became familiar with his own instrument panel, he could quickly scan it by looking only at the large markings and ignoring the small numbers or printing to decide if all was functioning properly. This could usually be done with the large peripheral field.

Many types of targets for training can be found around the home. Walking and bicycling offer good opportunities to employ these Bioptic training tehniques.

In the opinion of the author, many people with congenital low vision actually must learn to *see* when they get a Bioptic. The mirage effect of pavement which is off in the distance and appears wet is a common phenomenon often observed by normally sighted people. When the author first received his Bioptic, he had to learn that this effect was a mirage since he had never seen it before. Now with no corrective lenses at all and with no change in acuity he is able to notice this same phenomenon. It is evident that he could always see this mirage but was unaware of its presence because the brain could not interpret it. It is probable, therefore, that the increased visual resolution offered by the Bioptic teaches the brain how better to interpret visual stimuli even when the Bioptic is not being worn.

Professional Evaluation

VII. The assessment and evaluation of the person with low vision for the driving task should be completely in the hands of the professional in this area, namely, the Motor Vehicle examiners. If possible it is recommended that all visually handicapped persons pass their road competency test with one of several specially selected driving analysts employed by the Department of Motor Vehicles in that state. The theory provides that these few professionals will become skilled in evaluating low vision drivers and that there will be more standardization of expectations in performance.

In talking with several driver's license examiners in Massachusetts and California it was concluded that a comprehensive road test of at least one hour be given each low vision driver. This test would include all types of driving conditions, city streets, rural roads, freeways, and mountain hills and curves. The type of driving most often done by the prospective low vision driver would be stressed. If restrictions were to be imposed, the examiner would get a good idea as to the nature and extent of such restrictions in such a test.

All examiners interviewed stated that the low vision driver was evaluated in the same terms as any normally sighted driver. However, several critical areas singled out for special attention with low vision drivers were the following.

1. Speed control and braking time were noted. If the driver slammed on his brakes a half block from a red light, the examiner would assume that either the driver did not see the light or had judged the distance improperly.
2. Judging distances and widths of other objects was noted.
3. Steering around corners and curves, i.e. if the driver stayed in the center of his lane, was observed.
4. Use of mirrors to account for things happening in back of the driver, to scan head movements and eye movements, and to discern what was going on in front of the driver was noted.

Results

VIII. Can a person with a visual loss safely operate a motor vehicle? This is a question pondered by many at this point.

The first driver to obtain a legal driver's license using a Bioptic telescopic system was one of Korb's patients who received the license in 1967 in Massachusetts. There are now over twenty states and hundreds of licensed drivers who accept this aid as valid for passing the eye test and operating a motor vehicle. Unfortunately there are not any published statistical studies concerning the driving safety records of these individuals. However, statistics are often misleading. There had been no fatalities involving low vision drivers until October of 1973 when a deaf, blind pedestrian walked into the side of a moving truck and was killed. Had a normally sighted individual been at the wheel, the result would no doubt have been the same. On December 27, 1973, however, there was a second fatality in which the low vision driver was apparently at fault, although the facts for this case have not been disclosed.

The following few statistics are those compiled by Korb[1] in Massachusetts and are the only ones currently available. These statistics are from June 1, 1967 to May 31, 1973.

TABLE XXIII-I
POPULATION OF LOW VISION DRIVERS

SEX	NO. OF DRIVERS
MALE	117
FEMALE	11
TOTAL	128
AGE RANGE	
UNDER 21	12
22 to 34	19
35 to 50	38
51 to 66	44
over 66	9
MONTHS OF OPERATION	
6 to 12	8
13 to 23	20
24 to 35	64
36 to 47	23
48 to 59	7
over 60	6
PREVIOUS DRIVING EXPERIENCE OF THE SAMPLE	
Previous experience	97
No previous experience	15
Status in doubt	16
SAFETY RECORD 6/1/67 to 5/31/73	
Low vision operators	128
Man-years of driving	341
Accidents involving low vision driver regardless of fault	5
Accidents where low vision driver at fault	1

By calculation, for every 68.2 man-years of driving, a low vision driver can be predicted to be involved in an accident. Actually in the current statistics (Table XXIII-I), for every 341 man-years of driving, a low vision driver was involved in an accident which was his fault. The probability of this favorable distribution appearing by chance is 1 in 5,000. This compares very favorably to the general population of drivers for Massachusetts for this same time period in which the man-years of driving for an *at fault* accident for the general public was 17.6 man-years.

These are merely the highlights and a summary of one particular sample of low vision drivers. Because this group had a superior record as compared to the average driver, we cannot imply that all visually handicapped drivers will drive more safely than the general public, nor does it mean that everyone with low vision who is given a Bioptic will be a good driver. It can be concluded, however, that responsible individuals with low vision can very successfully use the Bioptic telescope as a low vision aid to assist them in operating a motor vehicle safely. The eye specialist should make the initial judgment as to whether the patient meets the visual prerequisites. The specialists may even wish to ride with the low vision driver before the patient is granted a license, but the final judgement of competency should be left up to the Division of Motor Vehicles since it is better qualified to make such a decision.

REFERENCES

1. Korb, Donald R.: Preparing the visually handicapped person for motor vehicle operation. *Am J Optom,* 47(8): 619-28, 1970.
2. Kelleher, Dennis K., Mehr, Edwin B., and Hirsch, Monroe J.: Motor vehicle operation by a patient with low vision; a case report. *Am J Optom* 48(9): 773-76, 1971.

· CHAPTER XXIV ·

A Cautionary View of Driving With Telescopes

George O. Hellinger

Introduction

IN NEW York State a motor vehicle operator is required to have 20/40 vision in only one eye. The other may have any degree of vision and may even be totally blind. When the required vision is not obtainable with standard spectacles, some practitioners have resorted to the use of telescopic devices to attain the required visual acuity for their patients.

While these devices *do* permit the operator to obtain passable chart-measured acuities, there are certain elements introduced that require our attention and discussion.

Considerations in Use of Telescopic Devices

It is recommended that the telescopic device be placed in the upper portion of the carrier lens so that the driver can look through it by adjustment of his head when he wishes to see distant objects. At all other times his view should be through the carrier lens or in a flip-up type frame arrangement as illustrated in Figure XXIV-I. This, of course, raises two questions.

1. While the operator is fixing his gaze through the telescopic portion, can he perceive any stimuli from the surrounding field in proper perspective, and can the person react rapidly to those stimuli which are not within of the field of view of the telescopic field?
2. What about the driver's vision when looking through the carrier lens? The answer might be as follows. We can assume

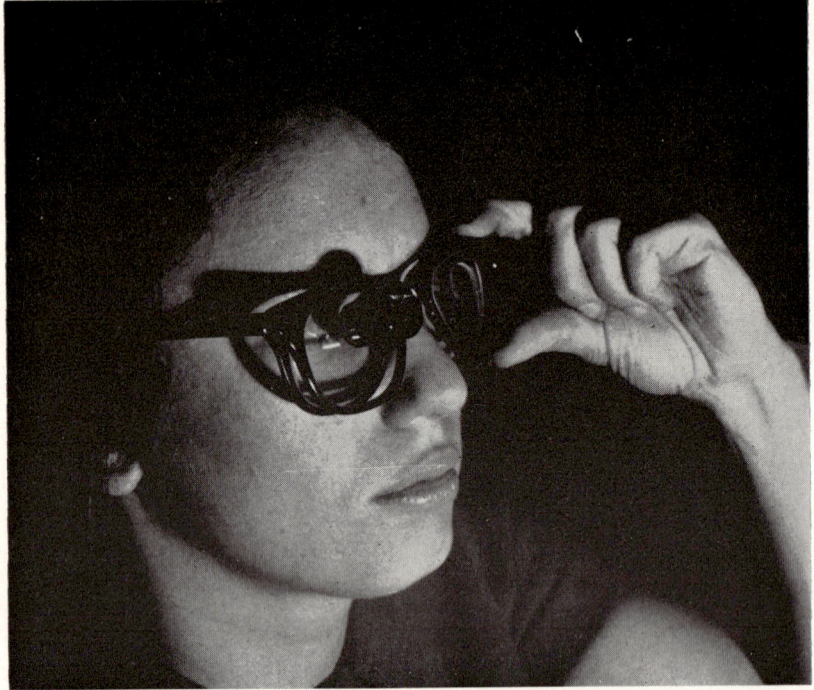

Figure XXIV-1. Telescopic arrangement with flip-up frame.

that the corrected vision with a standard lens is below 20/40; hence, the requirement for a telescopic arrangement.

It would be safe to assume that if a person required a 2.2x telescope, vision without the telescope, at best, would be only 20/100. If a 3.0x telescope is required to obtain 20/40, the original vision will be 20/200.

The visual field is an important factor in safe driving. Normally one depends on having an unobstructed peripheral field. If a driver looks through a wide angle 2.2x telescope, the central field is a magnified view of 17°. If a standard 3.0x telescope is needed, the field is only 8°.

So now we have a driver *legally blind* by virtue of *acuity* through the spectacle carrier lens and *legally blind* by virtue of the *field restriction* through the telescope. This creates what would seem to be a great hazard, especially if the operator has only one usable eye.

Recently, several articles have appeared in which the subjects who were using telescopic devices have been unusually cooperative and capable of adjustment to this unusual situation. It is conceivable that, if these telescopic spectacles become a standard operating procedure without stringent regulations, some individuals who are not as competent might be less able to cope with the actual driving situation. Or if these spectacles were to be used exclusively as a *spotting system,* i.e. for identifying travel signs, exit signs, what is to prevent a driver with 20/800 vision from using a small 8x (Zeiss) telescope mainly as an expedient method of passing the present motor vehicle requirements?

It is also important to consider the difference between city and rural driving when evaluating an individual who will be handling his vehicle in either or both situations.

Unfortunately, New York's state motor vehicle law does not require field-of-vision testing. It must be apparent that good peripheral vision is an essential prerequisite and should be tested in all cases applying for special licensing.

Another question to resolve is, Can the driver use the rearview mirror or the outside rearview mirror effectively?

The physician, the optometrist, or the Motor Vehicle Bureau can issue a certificate which states that the patient has the vision required by law on renewal of license; but is the examiner required to state that a special device is being used, or can he quite truthfully say the corrected visual acuity is 20/40 or better with corrective glasses? Would the examiner at the Motor Vehicle Bureau also merely indicate the need for *corrective* spectacles?

If this is so, will the driver end up with no restrictions on his license beyond corrective spectacles? How about night driving? Will these spectacles present a further hazard? The National Safety Council reports that 55 percent of all traffic fatalities occur after dark when only 33 percent of the driving is done. In addition, should there be any speed restrictions for this group?

Summary

At best, the use of these devices presents many problems that should be carefully evaluated, catalogued, and studied so that conditions

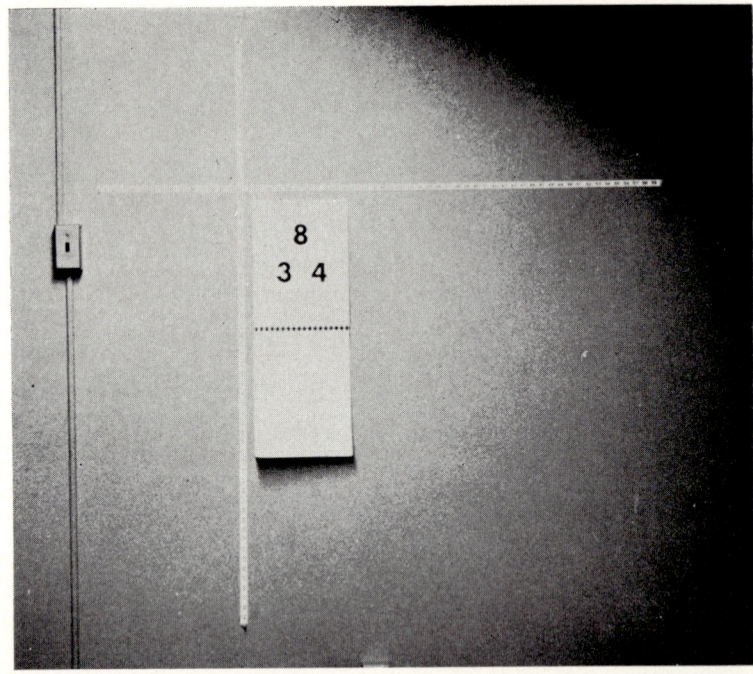

Figure XXIV-2. Normal field of view.

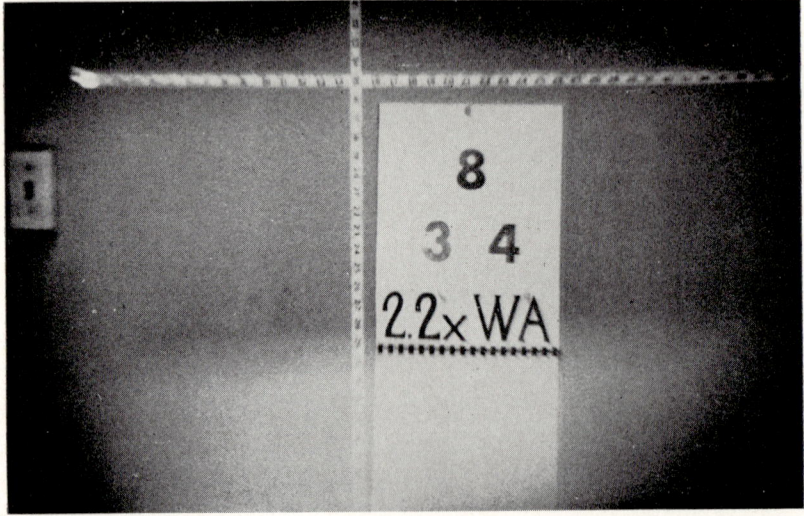

Figure XXIV-3. Field of view seen through 2.2x wide-angle Designs for Vision telescope is 17°.

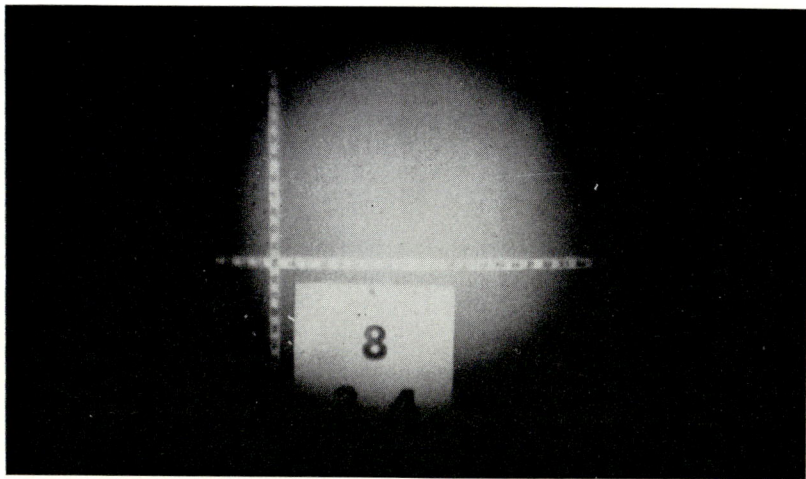

Figure XXIV-4. A 3.0x telescope reduces the field to 8°.

under which such devices are used, if allowed at all, are well controlled and strict. Limitations should be well outlined and understood by doctors, drivers, and the Department of Motor Vehicles so that no decision has to be made by guesswork or wishful thinking.

· CHAPTER XXV ·
Operational Limitations of Driving With Telescopes

Arthur H. Keeney
and Sidney Weiss

Statistical Examples

Traffic fatalities for the first six months of 1973 totalled 26,500, the highest number of traffic deaths ever recorded for the first half of any year in the history of the United States according to the National Safety Council.[1]

Traffic deaths for the first six months of 1973 increased by 2 percent over the total for the first six months of 1972.[2]

These statistics point out the need for strict enforcement of visual as well as other physical and mental standards for auto drivers' licenses and renewals.

In Pennsylvania, 20/40 in the better eye with best correction is the minimal standard for unrestricted driving. Restriction to daylight driving is placed on those who have been reported to have poor night vision or optimally corrected vision at the level of 20/50 to 20/70 using both eyes together. In 1970, the Medical Advisory Board recommended horizontal form-field requirements of 140°, but this has not yet been implemented. This can be met by the one-eyed driver. The 20/40 level of minimal acuity is selected because the lettering on freeway control signs is sized to be read by a driver with acuity of at least 20/40 at usual roadway speeds and normal weather conditions and is sufficient to make appropriate vehicular maneuvers.

Massachusetts, New Hampshire, California, Maine, North Carolina, and Florida have granted motor vehicle driver's licenses to people who can pass the vision test with telescopic spectacles. The telescopic spectacles used for this purpose are named Bioptic because the telescope is placed in the upper part of the spectacle lens, and permits vision through the spectacle lens by changing fixation.

Recommendations Against Telescopic Devices

Koetting[3] in 1969 advised against the use of telescopic lenses for motor vehicle operation.

Korb[4] reported his experience on twenty low vision patients who were licensed in Massachusetts to drive a motor vehicle. He recommended the following criteria for motor vehicle operation by visually handicapped persons utilizing telescopic systems.

1. Visual acuity with the telescopic system must meet minimal state requirements.
2. The visual field should be within normal limits when measured by standard methods.
3. The telescopic unit should be designed to be available for use with minimal head movements but when not in use should not impair the visual field utilized in driving.
4. The individual should undergo a minimum of two months of adaptation with the custom-designed telescopic spectacles.
5. An individual's road competency test should be made by the motor vehicle examining body of the particular state while the individual is wearing and using the telescopic prosthesis.
6. The telescopic prosthesis should be worn at all times when the individual is operating a motor vehicle.
7. Operation at night, on expressways, and under extreme conditions should be considered on an individual basis.

Korb further stated that adaptation to Bioptic systems is not accomplished without difficulty and that a multitude of problems have been encountered by subjects during adaptation.

On attempted use of the telescopic spectacles for driving, we have found the following problems.

1. There is a difficulty in maintaining the head in slight extension in order to see through the spectacle lens portion of the system.
2. There is difficulty of shifting rapidly from the magnification of the telescopic unit to the unmagnified image of the carrier lens.
3. The ring scotoma surrounding the magnified field presents a

significant jack-in-the-box hazard especially when passing and at intersections.
4. Vibration of the motor vehicle diminishes visual acuity, especially that acuity obtained through magnification.
5. There is a need to maintain reference points in the magnified field. Some portion of the automobile must be retained in the magnified field to reduce spatial disorientation.
6. It is impossible to use side and rearview mirrors when looking through the telescope.*

Fonda's[5] experience was personal and based upon six patients on whom visual fields were plotted on a tangent screen through the Bioptic telescope. His curiosity was aroused by the statements that the monocular field of vision for a 2.2x telescope was 22°, the binocular field 35°, and the ring scotoma 8° in width.†

With the telescope fitted at a vertex distance of 12mm, Fonda reported the peripheral field to be unrestricted; but the central magnified field for his dominant left eye was 7°, and the binocular central field was also 7°.

The ring scotoma extended 12° beyond this magnified central field in all directions. He states, "I was as conscious of the size of the ring scotoma as I was of the narrow field." In addition to these disadvantages, the telescopic system gave illusory movement in the opposite direction with any movement of the head.

The wearer of the Bioptic looks through the spectacle lenses continually except when he wants to spot a sign or car at a distance; then he tilts his head and looks through the telescope. People who wear the Bioptic state that they are useful for this purpose on a highway but not in the city where the distances are not great and the traffic is heavy.

The principal purpose of the telescope is to pass the driver's test and to some extent to read signs. Since the wearer does not use the telescope while driving except for spotting signs at a distance, he is still for all practical purposes driving with his low vision.

* This last problem is not substantiated by the editor's personal experience.
† Designs for Vision manufactures three 2.2x telescopes. The specifications revised in 1974 for monocular fields are: Bioptic I 12°, Bioptic II 10°, Wide-angle Bioptic 17°.

Summary

In summary, the technical objective of passing a state visual acuity test is negated by the following several major operational limitations.

1. Size distortion or nearness illusion leads to poor distance judgement.
2. A major ring scotoma intrudes on the visual field.
3. There is a need for maintaining extension of the head for looking through the spectacle lens.
4. There is illusory movement of objects in opposite direction to any head movement.
5. Resolution decay is induced by vibration.

REFERENCES

1. *Accident Facts, 1974 Edition,* National Safety Council, p. 50.
2. Ibid, 1973 Edition, p. 50.
3. Koetting, R. A.: The simplified approach to low vision. *Journal of the American Optometric Association, 40(8):* 851-53, 1969.
4. Korb, D. R.: Preparing the visually handicapped person for motor vehicle operation. *Am J Optom, 47(8)*: 619-28, 1970.
5. Fonda, G.: Personal communication, 1973.

· CHAPTER XXVI ·
Discussion of Driving Criteria
Alan H. Barnert

A Summarization of Differing Conclusions

As was foreseen, we have no agreement on the answers to the questions, although we do have a large area of agreed-upon facts among the differing conclusions. Let us first summarize what has been said and then see wherein we agree and disagree.

Drs. Newman and Tallman are both from very different areas of the country; yet, each reports very similar experiences and favorable conclusions about telescopes for driving. They each note the economic and sociological need to drive a car, the lack of a scientific basis for the present driving requirements, and the variability between state requirements. They both suggest strict criteria for selection of possible candidates for driving with telescopes, rigorous training, and special road testing. Their criteria are similar to each other and to Korb's criteria[1], and they each report favorable accident experience with their own groups of drivers.

Drs. Hellinger and Weiss are also from different cities, and have more discouraging reports. They emphasize such disadvantages of telescopes as their small field of vision, the ring scotoma, the loss of time in switching from the telescope to the carrier, and, in general, the danger to the public. Dr. Hellinger points out, however, that until the term *corrective lenses* is clarified, such patients actually meet the New York state requirements for driving. Dr. Weiss showed us a movie to demonstrate the loss of field when using a telescopic system.

Dr. Scott, who has been unable to obtain departmental release for publication of his paper, has acquainted us with the problems encountered by the agency which actually has to make the decisions. He stresses the state agency's problems, the lack of data, the importance of driving to the potential drivers, the responsibility to the public, the pressures from organizations both outside and inside the government, from private interested individuals, and from their lawyers, and the public relations problem of allowing *blind* drivers on the road. Whether these drivers be called legally blind, partially blind, or partially sighted, one fact is certain: like all other drivers, sooner or later they will be involved in accidents and fatalities.

Areas of Agreement

Let us now summarize what we know and what we do not know, and let us try to reach a conclusion. We agree that the state requirements are varied and that some of them, e.g. depth perception, seem unnecessary. It would seem preferable to have them not only more uniform but more flexible in the areas of visual acuity and peripheral fields. We are all aware that driving is an important function to most adults and that numbers of persons who cannot meet the visual requirements can be made to do so with a special telescope. These telescopic spectacles have either a 2.2x, 3x, or (rarely) 4x telescopic unit mounted in the upper portion of the carrier. It is possible to adapt to this set-up and drive with it. To date, a reasonably large group of people have been driving with these aids, and the number of accidents has been reasonably low.[1] There have been accidents, however; but the experience has not been extensive enough yet to permit evaluation of the factors which were involved in the accidents. The drivers up to now have been carefully selected and carefully fitted and trained by a small group of practitioners.[2] A larger, more general group of drivers fitted with telescopes would presumably not meet the strict requirements of selection, training, and testing for the present group.

Recommendations

In light of the preceding information, the author has arrived at the following conclusions.[*]

1. It seems clear that the various States should reexamine their

---

[*] These are the author's and editor's personal conclusions, not the position of either The Lighthouse or the panel; and they may change as more facts come in.

requirements for driver's licenses with a view towards making them both uniform and more in line with what is known about the factors in driving, i.e. add field requirements where they do not exist and eliminate unnecessary requirements. This is for general requirements and has nothing to do with telescopes.

2. There is a misconception which is fairly widespread and has caused a good deal of opposition to the very idea of *driving with telescopes*. This misconception is as follows, "A restricted field of vision is very disabling, even for walking and certainly for driving. The field of vision through a telescope is very restricted. Therefore a telescope is not suited for driving." This ignores the fact that driving with the telescopic glasses, involves using vision through the spectacle portion, *not* through the telescope. The telescope is used only for *spotting* highway signs, street names, and so on. It is true but irrelevant that it would be well-nigh impossible to use the telescope itself for basic driving vision.

Perhaps one other point should be mentioned here. Everyone has a gut reaction against lowering visual requirements for driving, especially to the point of allowing for *blind* drivers. But decisions should be made on the facts gathered from experience, not on first reactions.

3. It also seems clear that we need much more knowledge about basic factors in driving such as the relationship of visual acuity to detecting clues in driving. Much more research should be done on this most important subject.

4. With respect to telescopes, our recommendations are the following. Do *not* change any laws yet, but continue the informal system which is in effect today. This allows us to learn the pros and cons gradually and to sharpen our views on requirements, criteria for selection, and safety statistics during a period when only a few carefully selected and observed drivers are on the road.

A change in the laws to legalize telescopes for driving would have many disadvantages. There are not enough facts known to permit a rational set of requirements, and, if they are either too strict or too lenient, they will not be of much value. Again, once telescopes are legislated as permissible, it would be almost impossible to take away licenses even if it later turns out that they are undesirable.

The present, informal system may be the best one for an evolving situation, and it does contain a good system of controls based on the criteria of the prescribing doctor and the discretion of the motor vehicle department which is observing the candidate.

It will be interesting to see what the future brings.

REFERENCES

1. Korb, Donald R.: Preparing the visually handicapped person for motor vehicle operation. *Am J Optom,* 47(8): 619-28, 1970.
2. Kelleher, Dennis K., Mehr, Edwin B., and Hirsch, Monroe, J.: Motor vehicle operation by a patient with low vision: a case report. *Am J Optom,* 48(9): 773-76, 1971.

· SECTION EIGHT ·
Models of Low Vision Clinics

· CHAPTER XXVII ·

Low Vision Clinics: The Need, The Organization, The Manpower

RANDALL T. JOSE

Manpower Problems

THERE ARE numerous publications which point out the manpower shortage in the eye care field today.[1,2,3,4] These figures indicate a definite need for increasing the manpower supply in this vital area of health care. One has only to try to make an appointment for an eye examination to realize how accurate these figures are. There are no published statistics on the availability of services in the specialized area of care for the partially sighted. This is an unique population which is extremely difficult to reach or even define. They have many vision and vision related problems that the typical eye practitioner does not have the knowledge, facilities, or time to care for properly. Many clinics and/or practitioners will attempt to work with these people, but they are only able to provide a small part of the total vision rehabilitation program needed.

Reasons for this lack of services include the low emphasis on this aspect of care in the professional educational programs; poor financial returns for participation in this area of care; high time investment necessary in working with these patients; and the seeming lack of success that practitioners often associate with the prescribing of optical aids. As a result of these factors, it is estimated that less than 1 percent of eye care facilities provide their patients with a program of vision enhancement through the use of specialized optical and nonoptical aids and services.[5]

Organizational Problems

Even this situation would be tolerable if a proper referral system were utilized in the professions. Unfortunately, many practitioners are still not convinced of the advantages of a rigorous vision rehabilitation training program with optical aids for improving a patient's ability to function visually. For the most part, their experiences with this type of care are usually from a *cafeteria* style clinic in which a patient picks out his own magnifier with minimum professional guidance. The doctor may have provided a more sophisticated examination procedure in which a more complicated prescription was designed (usually in spectacle form) but inadequate training and follow-up programs for the patient were supplied. These programs usually suffer a 40 percent failure rate and are remembered more than the success cases. They cannot see the advantage of exposing themselves or their patients to the frustration of a long examination procedure and expensive lenses and then have the patient not able to use them. It is this, "They will only put them in the top drawer of their bureau," attitude that keeps many practitioners from referring their low vision patients for proper care. They just do not recognize the significance that a good program in low vision care can have for their patients. A second problem exists in that there are relatively few clinics or practitioners to whom one can refer patients. If we stipulate that referrals be only to comprehensive programs of care, we are even more drastically limiting the referral sources available to the practitioners. Statistics being gathered by the National Society for the Prevention of Blindness indicate that there are less than two hundred low vision clinics of one sort or another scattered throughout the United States.[5] We will not belabor the point further. It's quite obvious that there is a definite manpower shortage in the area of vision care for the partially sighted. As with the manpower shortage in the eye care field in general, this shortage can be remedied through some very specific programs of paraprofessional assistance and development of many well located interdisciplinary clinics.

Population Needs

To really understand the problem of needs, we must now look at the population that these clinic facilities must serve. The statistics on the extent of legal blindness in the United States are confusing at best. It is estimated that of the approximately 500 thousand to one million legally blind persons in the United States today,[6,7] as many as 75 percent to 85 percent of them could be helped with some form of optical or nonoptical aid.[8,9] Yet, it is felt that only one half of these people are receiving services.[10,11] If this is the case with the more easily identifiable population of legally blind*, then one can imagine the difficulty in defining a population of partially sighted or visually handicapped. There are no definitely accepted administrative standards to guide one in making a good epidemiological study of this group of people.[12] For our purposes I would like to offer a definition of the partially sighted. Dr. Edwin Mehr, School of Optometry, University of California at Berkeley states that, "... a partially sighted person is one who with conventional corrections is not able to perform vision tasks needed for vocational, avocational, or social needs." This definition probably closely reflects the criteria established by the National Health Survey in their study of visual impairments. Specifically, they registered as "severely visually impaired" anyone who could not read a newspaper with his present correction. From this rather flexible and poorly controlled criteria, they managed to come up with some five million people whom we could consider partially sighted. It is disheartening to reflect on the possibility that only half of this population is receiving substantial benefit from a low vision program.

Still another problem exists in familiarizing this population and the various professionals that serve this population with the existence of low vision programs. Many geriatric patients are huddled in their homes and living like vegetables because they have had a severe loss of vision and have been told to go home and learn to live with it. Learning to live with a severe vision loss is not something one just picks up, especially if one is seventy years of age. Careful counseling, guidance, and training are needed to make these persons independent and self-sufficient.

As programs are developed to acquaint the public with low vision care programs, and as in-service type training seminars are used to

---

* Legal blindness is an administrative definition which indicates that a person is eligible for blind services if his best corrected acuity with conventional lenses in the better eye is 20/200 or worse. A field loss which restricts peripheral vision to 20° or less is also defined as legal blindness.

acquaint professionals working with the partially sighted with low vision care, we can expect an increase in the percentage of people receiving these services.

More and more agencies are changing the emphasis of their program to reflect the needs of the partially sighted clients instead of the totally blind.[13] This change in attitude will result in a greater demand for eye care professionals to work in comprehensive vision care clinical programs and will foster a renewed interest among private practitioners to offer a solid program of diagnosis, treatment, and training for their partially sighted patients. This, of course, leads us right back to our present problem of manpower shortage. We are not successfully meeting the present needs of this population: it is going to be a tremendous challenge to build competent programs of care for this expected expanded population.

REFERENCES

1. National Center for Health Statistics: *Optometrists Employed in Health Services, United States-1968,* DHEW Publication, (HSM) 73-1803, Vital and Health Statistics, ser. 14, no. 8, March, 1973.
2. National Center for Health Statistics: *Ophthalmology Manpower: Characteristics of Clinical Practice, United States-1968,* DHEW Publication, (HSM) 73-1802, Vital and Health Statistics, ser. 14, no. 7, March, 1973.
3. *A Demographic Study and Analysis of the Optometric Profession in the United States.* Chicago, Professional Press, Inc., January, 1972.
4. Peters, Hank B., and Kleinstein, Robert: The availability of optometric manpower in California, 1968-2000. *Am J Optom, 46(4),* 1969.
5. *Directory of Low Vision Aids Facilities in the United States.* New York, National Society for the Prevention of Blindness, 1973-1974.
6. *Estimated Statistics on Blindness and Vision Problems-NSPB Factbook.* New York, National Society for the Prevention of Blindness, 1966.
7. Scott, Robert: *The Making of Blind Men.* New York, Russell Sage. 1969.
8. Jose, Randall: Getting started in the low vision field. *Optometric Weekly,* March 20, 1969.
9. Jose, Randall: Optical aids: an interdisciplinary prescription. *New Outlook for the Blind, 67:* 1, 1973.
10. Organization for Social and Technical Innovation, Inc.: *Blindness and Services to the Blind in the United States.* Massachusetts, OSTI Press, 1968.
11. American Foundation for the Blind: Policy statement on aging and visual

impairment. In *Regional Invitational Symposium on Attitudes on Blindness,* New York, June, 1972.
12. Riley, Leo H.: The Epidemiology of Partial Sight. *Am J Optom, 47*:(8), 1970.
13. Rosenbloom, Alfred A., Jr.: Subnormal vision aids. In Proceedings of the Thirty-First Convention of the American Association of Workers for the Blind, Chicago, July, 1957.

· CHAPTER XXVIII ·

A Low Vision Program in Rochester, New York

Ellis Gruber

Introduction

THE LIGHTHOUSE Low Vision Service should be congratulated on their 20th anniversary. It represents a milestone in the history of the art or science of low vision in this country.

The Lighthouse has not only been a shining beacon and a guiding light to thousands of low vision patients over these years but also to the many low vision centers which have more recently sprung up in many areas. Such a one is the Low Vision Center in Rochester, New York. It is hoped that those who do not have such a center available or those who are contemplating starting one will be helped and encouraged by knowing the history and progress of our program.

Phase One

The Rochester Low Vision Center has gone through three phases from its inception to the present day. The first phase took place in 1967 when the need was first established and the Low Vision Clinic was given a place at the Eye Department of the Strong Memorial Hospital, an affiliate of the University of Rochester School of Medicine and Dentistry. The staff at that time consisted of the author and one optician, and the equipment was contained in one small suitcase that the optician brought with him to the clinic which was held once a month. We had no secretary, no social worker, no prescreening, no follow-ups, no proper referrals, no money, no storage space, and no permanent location. We did expand, however, to the extent that the optician would bring three cases of equipment instead of one. After 1½ years I met with the director of the local Association for the Blind of Rochester and Monroe County who had no such service in his agency. He was very anxious for a low vision service to continue in the community. He was able to provide staff and some money for equipment. Neither of us wished to change the location of the clinic or to take it out of university sponsorship. It also served a useful purpose as a part of the resident training program. What we requested was a permanent room to call our own, but this was not forthcoming. Meanwhile, the Association for the Blind had commited themselves to provide a low vision examination as a part of their rehabilitation process.

Phase Two

So phase two began in October, 1969 when we moved temporarily and under Association auspices to a room in my office, where at least we had a permanent area and some storage space. We increased our staff to include a full-time social worker, a coordinator provided by the Association, and another three local ophthalmologists who rotated the clinics with me. Mrs. Margaret Sample, R.N. screened and interviewed all patients prior to their being seen in the clinic. She did follow-up visits in the homes of all patients who had been given an aid. We had a small inventory of aids in stock, so that we could give or loan an aid to many of the patients immediately. This provided a tremendous boost to the patients as they had the aid when they needed it most, directly after their low vision examination. We were really beginning to progress. Our service was made available regardless of age to all persons who had low but some measurable vision. Referrals came from many sources such as M.D.'s, opticians, eye clinics, nurses, the State Rehabilitation Counseling Service, friends, and patients themselves. We have had no liaison with optometrists to date; but we are hoping to include them to help in our clinic in the future, and they are another obvious source of referral. Besides serving our own county of Monroe, our service is also provided to five other counties; namely, Livingston, Ontario, Seneca, Wayne, and Yates in upstate New York.

Phase Three

I was never happy having the clinic in my office. I felt there was a reluctance among the ophthalmologists to refer their patients to another private office. When the time came in early 1972 for the Association for the Blind to move into its new quarters, it seemed like the ideal time to establish the permanent low vision clinic there.

So the third phase began in March, 1973 when the clinic moved from my office to the Association for the Blind. They bought and remodeled a large old building and gave us the space we needed. Three rooms were designed for our use; an office for the coordinator and a secretary, a room containing the larger aids and in which the optician could work with the patient, and a large examining room furnished with all the necessary ophthalmic equipment for a complete eye evaluation. This, for the first time, gave us all the facilities we needed.

One may wonder about the source of funds. They come from a variety of sources. Every patient seen is partially subsidized by the Association because the fees paid are less than expenses incurred. The Association is a part of the local Community Chest and receives a yearly grant from that source. The Rehabilitation Counseling Service pays for the patients on their state program. We are presently negotiating with Medicaid to pay for the aid. Private patients pay a fee similar to what they would pay at any medical office. There are also private donations given to the Association.

We have devised our own forms for history, for low vision exam, for requests from referring sources for past history, and for information to be returned to the referring source about visual acuity and the aids prescribed.

Community Programs

We have had two all-day work shops, one cosponsored by the Association for the Blind and the Rehabilitation Counseling Service and the New York State Commission for the Blind, and the other cosponsored by the Association and a local home for the aged. These workshops provide a most effective means of communicating with personnel from nursing homes, sanatoriums, institutions, homes for the aged, counselors, and social service workers. These professionals who deal with low vision patients on a day-to-day basis are most anxious to learn about the services available to the partially sighted, and they find it most helpful to hear about low vision problems, symptoms, the types of aids available and what the aids can be expected to accomplish. *It is very important to let all groups in the community know that low vision services are available and instruct them on how they can refer suitable patients there.*

Useful Aids

The aids we have found to be most useful are usually those that have been listed in other studies. Nothing can take the place of a good up-to-date refraction and the use of bifocals with high reading adds. Half-eye readers with base-in prism are very useful by themselves or worn over the patient's regular bifocals. The Ary Loupe which can be easily attached to the glasses over the better eye and flipped up and down at will is an inexpensive and useful aid. Hand magnifiers and stand magnifiers, especially the COIL series, are well liked by the patients. In the more powerful range are the folding pocket magnifiers of Bausch & Lomb. For distance vision, the 2.5x Selsi monocular telescope* has been found the most useful for spot checking the school board and street signs, and the best telescopic system appears to be the one obtainable from Designs for Vision of New York. Besides spectacles, almost thirty types of aids have been prescribed, and the most common ones used can be seen in Table XXVIII-I. In reviewing our last 250 patients we found that two hundred (80%) were given aids, and on follow-up we found that 150 (60%) were really helped by the aid.

Table XXVIII-II lists the ocular pathology that was found most commonly in 198 consecutive cases. By far the most frequent condition was macular degeneration followed by diabetic retinopathy, optic atrophy, and chorioretinitis.

Program Problems

Our failures have been due mainly to lack of motivation on the part of the patient and occasionally to an error in prescription or a change in the eye condition since the aid prescription, e.g. diabetic hemorrhage.

---

* The above aids are available from *Catalogue of Optical Aids,* rev. 3rd ed. New York, New York Lighthouse Low Vision Service, 1973.

TABLE XXVIII-I
TYPE, NUMBER, AND PERCENTAGE OF AIDS PRESCRIBED

Type of Aid		Number	Percentage
SPECTACLES		59	35.5
(includes regular bifocals, high add bifocals, and half eyes with base-in prism)			
TELESCOPES		37	22.0
Hand-held Monocular			
2.5x	24		
6.0x	2		
7.0x	1		
8.0x	5		
Spectacle			
Aloe 1.8x	1		
Designs for Vision			
2.2x	1		
Sport glasses 2.5x	2		
2.8x	1		
MAGNIFIERS, HAND HELD		20	12.2
Bausch and Lomb 4 D	2		
Chest magnifier 5 D	6		
McLeod 11 D	1		
COIL 20 D	4		
Bausch and Lomb 7x	2		
Bausch and Lomb 12x	5		
MAGNIFIERS, STAND		27	16.3
Bausch and Lomb			
Illuminated 4 D	2		
Luxo 3x	2		
Donegan Paper Weight 5x	2		
COIL 20 D	6		
COIL 29 D	15		
LOUPES		20	12.2
Telesite	4		
Ary	15		
Carton Binocular	1		
CLOSED CIRCUIT TELEVISION		3	1.8
Optiscope	1		
Visualtek	2		

Some of our initial problems were due to lack of space, staff and equipment. Others have been the inability of the patient to buy the aid because of the high cost involved, and we have always kept the economic factor in mind and used aids that are less expensive without sacrificing quality. Also, lack of acceptance by the medical and optometric community had to be overcome. This took time and needed open communication and some education. It has been

TABLE XXVIII-II
OCULAR PATHOLOGY

Rating	Primary Diagnosis	Number of Patients
1	Macular Degeneration	67
2	Diabetic Retinopathy Including Proliferans and Hemorrhages	30
3	Optic Atrophy	27
4	Myopic Degeneration	12
5	Chorioretinitis Including Histoplasmosis and Circinate Retinitis	11
6	Cataract————Congenital	8
	————Senile	2
7	Glaucoma————Congenital	3
	————Chronic Simple	6
8	Retrolental Fibroplasia	8
9	Retinitis Pigmentosa	5
10	Congenital Coloboma	3
11	Microphthalmos	3
12	Corneal Opacification	3
13	Keratoconus	2
14	Uveitis	2
15	Retinal Detachment	2
16	Vitreous Hemorrhage	1
17	Interstitial Keratitis	1
18	Albinism	1
19	Aphakia	1

planned to invite each of these groups to the center to show them what we have to offer. In the final analysis it will be the patient results which will tell the real story. I would like to relate two examples which will illustrate this.

Case Examples

About three years ago a well-known local ophthalmologist informed me that he had heard about our low vision clinic, and he wondered what we could do that he could not. I answered that there was really nothing except that perhaps we had more aids than he had available in his office. He reluctantly sent a patient to us shortly after, and she was sent back to him a much happier patient with an aid which gave her 20/20 and J#1 vision. I think that was enough to convince him of the value of a low vision clinic.

The second case is that of a thirty-one-year-old lady seen quite recently. She had been through the eye department of the University on numerous occasions over the last 3½ years and had been examined by many doctors. Her best vision was 20/200 and J#7 in each eye.

On looking through her record it was obvious that the diagnosis was not clear and that it was an unusual case. It was concluded as being an achromatopsia or a hypoplasia of the macula. The point to be made here is important. From the patient's point of view the diagnosis is not important. What is important is that something practical must be done for her. Not only was the New York State Mandatory Eye Medical Report never sent in for her case, but in 3½ years she had *never* been given a trial with a low vision aid. I gave her an 8x Selsi telescope which gives her 20/25 vision and a 20-diopter COIL stand magnifier with which she reads J#2, and for the first time in years she is able to function reasonably well and is a much happier person for it. The conclusion to be drawn from the above is not to get lost in diagnostics because it is purely academic and does not help the patient. The main concern is to try visual aids on all patients with poor vision and not lose sight of the forest because of the trees.

One other problem for patients under the State Rehabilitation program is the withholding of approval for the purchase of the aid until the whole data on the patient has been accumulated and sent in at the same time. If there are other services being given to the patient as is usually the case, all the information must be assembled in one package; thus, there can be long delays in getting approval for the aid. By this time the patient's stimulus, interest, and motivation created by the low vision exam have often been diminished.

The ophthalmologist should never lose sight of the fact that he has not just a pair of eyes under his care but a total person. Visual aids are only one part of the rehabilitation of a visually handicapped person. Other parts of the rehabilitation process include such things as physical fitness, general health, vocational training, mobility, homemaking, counseling, educational programs, recreation, placement, and communication, e.g. writing, telephoning, typing, talking books and tapes, and braille. Any or all of these may be very important to the individual. Low vision patients should be given the opportunity to try low vision aids, and we should not prejudge the probable success or failure for improved vision merely by observing the patient's visual acuity. It is often amazing how low the visual acuity can be and yet how well the patients can perform if given the chance, especially on reading and close work. The formulas for estimating what strength of aid is needed for a given visual acuity should only be used as a guide. The formula may be useful, but, practically, if the case seems hopeless I would recommend that formulas be forgotten and every patient be given the opportunity to try some aids.

Summary

In summary then, what have we accomplished in Rochester in the last six years? Since starting with one small suitcase of low vision aids we now have a complete center with excellent staff, facilities, and equipment to provide help for the low vision patient who must learn to use what vision he has left, optimally within his ability. The patient has the opportunity under professional guidance and encouragement to try various visual aids in an environment especially designed for his problem. This provides a service which is not possible in the routine clinical practice of the average ophthalmologist, not necessarily due to his lack of ability but due to the lack of necessary equipment and, above all, due to the lack of time which is required.

Most patients derive some benefit from attending the clinic, if not from an actual aid then perhaps from the advice and suggestions he receives about the best use of the vision he has, types of lighting that should be used, and availability of non-optical aids such as large print books, large telephone dials, ruled paper, check books and stencils. Perhaps the patient is helped just from knowing that someone who really understands and cares about his problem is trying to help him. It is of great benefit to the patient to be given the aid immediately from our inventory (a common occurrence) and to know that he may come back at any time to try any aid under the guidance of Mrs. Sample. Such a service is certainly unique in our area.

I hope that this chapter explaining the local low vision program in Rochester will encourage those centers which are just beginning to forge ahead and will stimulate those areas in which there is no such service available to low vision patients to start one. If we can do it, you can. It will be most rewarding and will provide a very worthwhile service to a segment of our patient population which has been pushed aside and neglected for so long.

CHAPTER XXIX

The Vision Rehabilitation Clinic at Boston University Medical Center

THE ROLE OF THE OPHTHALMOLOGIST

Carter B. Tallman

Introduction

At the present time, we are seeing approximately five-hundred new patients per year; and, since the onset of the clinic in 1968, we have seen more than one thousand new patients (as of 1973).

The goals of the program are basically the following four.

1. To enable each patient to attain maximum use of his visual capacities so that his life may continue as normally and productively as possible; in other words, if possible, to remain independent.
2. To provide special training in vision rehabilitation to residents in ophthalmology and students of optometry, and to provide field work experience for graduate students in social work and rehabilitation counseling.
3. To conduct an educational program to increase understanding among eye care professionals and the public. I think this is exceedingly important and is one of the areas in which we have to work harder. We must get the message to the eye care professionals and the public about what a visually handicapped person needs and what he can and cannot do once he has been given adequate rehabilitation services.
4. To engage in research and development of new devices and techniques to allow the patient more effective use of his limited vision.

The following is a profile of the Vision Rehabilitation Clinic at

Boston University Medical Center; so, in essence, you will recognize us when you see us.

We work as a team consisting of the patient, social worker, optometrist, ophthalmologist, public and private agencies, psychiatrist, peripatologist, and special education teacher. Everybody works together with and for the patient.

In our clinic the same optometrist or ophthalmologist and the same social worker see the patient on each visit. Maintaining this same team on each visit is important in order to establish trust and rapport with the patient and in order to understand fully the patient's needs and goals.

Our goal is to make the patient as independent as he desires. We recognize that some patients do not want to be independent: some are happy in their symbiotic relationship with someone else.

We have a task oriented rehabilitation approach, that is, the patient tells us what it is that he wants to do. Then we try to provide the tools and the counseling that will enable him to perform these various tasks to his best ability.

Multiple Visits for A Single Fee

In order to remove monetary problems as much as possible (the elderly and children have less available funds, and the elderly require the most visits), we instituted a policy whereby the patient is seen in as many visits as is necessary for a single fee which covers a six-month period. The fee is sixty dollars. A patient is therefore seen in our clinic anywhere from two to six visits for one fee. If a patient is seen only once, there is a reduced fee. There is an additional fee for follow-up visits after the six-month period.

Loan System

I do not see how any clinic or any low vision practitioner can work without a loan system. I do not see how a doctor can determine which aid or high plus magnifying lens would work in the home or job situation of a patient unless the patient can be loaned a device. This device may not be exactly what would be prescribed in the end, but at least similar enough to introduce him to the multitude of problems that arise. The doctor and the patient can then begin to discover what is effective. It is interesting to note that not until the patient experiences some degree of success with one device does he begin to discuss other goals and problems that he previously thought were insolvable.

Trade-in System

This is a spin-off of the loan system. As you know, the diabetic patient is particularly prone to many fluctuations in visual acuity. If the patient's visual acuity changes after being prescribed a certain device, and if the device is in usable condition and is the type of aid that can be interchanged (such as high plus lenses), then the patient can trade it in without additional cost for another device which is appropriate and useful.

How We Achieve Our Goal of Independence

Adequate counseling of patients is essential. In order for the patient to become an active, participating member of the rehabilitation team, he must be informed. He must know his diagnosis and any known genetic factors so that he and his family can plan effectively for the future. He should know if he has multiple diagnoses such as macular degeneration and cataracts. He should have some idea as to what portion of his visual problem is related to each of these disease processes so that he understands that the glare problem is perhaps due to the cataract and the visual problem results from the macular degeneration. He must not become a misinformed patient who thinks he is on the cataract waiting list when, in fact, he will never have cataract surgery because of his retinal problems. We see patients who have retinitis pigmentosa and developing posterior subcapsular cataracts who become frightened because of a sudden change in visual acuity not related to the retinal disease but to the cataract changes. The patient fears that his doctor did not level with him and that he is, in fact, going to go suddenly and totally blind. When the patient understands his multiple diagnoses, he becomes more reassured and more trusting of the physician. We must let the patient know his prognosis whenever this is possible.

The patient should receive vocational counseling and training. My policy is to remain as unstructured as possible. I try to be as openminded and optimistic as possible: I believe that once a person is given a list of "jobs you can do," he immediately and automatically develops an extremely limited outlook. Instead, the subject should be approached from the point of view of "what jobs can't you do." This is a much smaller list. How do we know a patient's potential until we find out the patient's interests; until he tells us how far he has gone in the educational system; until the patient develops interests, drive, and motivation? Until he goes out and "hoofs it" by looking for a job, how does he know what vocational possibilities are available to him? When I counsel patients who are working with rehabilitation agencies in terms of getting a job, I tell the patient, "There is *nobody* who is going to look out for you as much as you yourself, and the responsibility for getting a job and an education rests with you just as much as it rests with your counselor." The agency may assist him; but, if he relies solely upon the agency, he is not taking advantage of the most important member of the team, himself.

Referral to appropriate agencies is mandatory, and communication with these agencies must ensue. Talk to the agency, write to the agency, visit the agency. Have the agency personnel come with their clients to the clinic. Go back to the agency and discuss with their field workers the general problems in the particular cases.

Follow-up is another step towards achieving our goal. We follow up on our patients in order to learn if we are helping them effectively. After the patient's last visit to our Clinic, we send him a questionnaire. The social workers make phone calls to patients whom they know should be followed. In one way or another we try to communicate with the patient.

Of course, in order for all of this to be effective, appropriate optical aids must be provided. The proper prescription of optical aids is not under discussion here; however, it should be stressed that multiple aids are usually necessary. A patient has many visual needs. These may include reading, writing, watching television, distance spotting, and typing. No single aid is appropriate for all these tasks.

The Role of the Ophthalmologist

At the Boston University Vision Rehabilitation Clinic the ophthalmologist and optometrist essentially perform in a similar manner. All patients must have a recent (within six months) ophthalmological report in the record prior to examination at the clinic. We recently instituted a policy whereby the senior resident in ophthalmology is scheduled to examine many new patients following their low vision examination by the optometrist. This is not the same resident rotating through the clinic who is referred to in the following section. This policy serves two purposes.

1. It provides a teaching case-load for the resident which has a high rate of interesting pathology, and it reminds the resident of the continuum of care which is so important. In other words, it is not an eyeball that is being treated but a patient with a variety of needs; and, until the doctor achieves maximum rehabilitation of the patient in his office, he has not completed his responsibility to his patient.
2. It affords the optometrist some support in providing counseling to the patient about prognosis and genetic factors. Also, any question of diagnosis can be answered at this time.

The ophthalmologist has the option of performing a complete ophthalmological examination on each new patient or on follow-up visits but, in fact, often does not do this because of the adequacy of the accompanying eye report. If the visual acuity and history indicates that there has been no change, then a full ophthalmological examination with dilated pupils is usually not done. This also emphasizes something that I feel is important; that is, we are part of a team with the referring physician.

Our responsibility to the physician includes a referral letter reporting to him what has been done for his patient and reassuring him that a referral is good medical practice if he does not care to do much of this in his own practice. I do not think low vision work should be done only in clinic situations, but, rather, the clinic should become a referral source for complicated low vision cases. We should continuously encourage eye care professionals in private practice to do some low vision work themselves, providing the patient does not need extensive teamwork.

Ophthalmology Residency Teaching

One resident rotates through our clinic for three months, one half of a day per week. All residents prior to their rotation in the Vision Rehabilitation Clinic are given an introductory series of lectures by the staff ophthalmologist, optometrist, and social worker. Each resident, prior to his low vision rotation, receives individual instruction in techniques, theory, clinical application, and specific record-keeping procedures. The resident observes and assists the staff ophthalmologist to perform low vision services until he is competent to do it alone. During this training period he is taught the specific uses of each type of low vision aid, from the simplest magnifier to the complex closed circuit television system. We give a bibliography of required reading to each resident.

The resident presents cases at our staff conferences, and he sees both new and follow-up patients. The time period for this rotation is not as long as it should be, but it is long enough to allow the young ophthalmologist to see a given patient for at least two or three visits. This is important in training doctors. Unless a doctor has responsibility for his own patients and follows up on them, he will not develop a real understanding of the problem.

Engineering and Development

We have had engineering help during different stages of our clinic. At one time we had an engineer, Phillip Davis, from the Massachusetts Commission for the Blind who worked closely with the Clinic and helped develop one of the first closed circuit television magnifying systems. At the present time we have the part-time help of another engineer. His most recent contribution was to electrify a Coil 3x and 4x hand magnifier which was previously battery powered. He also changed the bulb on these devices, increasing the bulb life fortyfold. This improvement and modification of optical aids is a small but important step. More work should be done on developing or adapting aids specifically for the needs of the partially sighted.

Summary

Without the tools or the hardware, that is, without the optical and nonoptical aids, we would not be able to do the job. However, these tools are only the means and not the end with which we help individuals. It is the whole person, not the eye or the vision, with whom we join to develop a rehabilitation program.

THE ROLE OF THE SOCIAL WORKER

Dagmar B. Friedman

Introduction

The social worker helps each patient understand his visual problems as they relate to his needs and life-style. The social worker explains clinic procedures to each patient and his family and begins the exploration of the patient's problems as they relate to his loss of vision. The effectiveness of patient care is often dependent on how well the social worker pulls together with the patient and his family the services from our clinic, from the referring physician, and from other community agencies.

The social worker carefully notes the age of the patient, the circumstances surrounding the onset of visual loss, the duration of loss, and the severity of loss; and notes what the patient knows about his eye disease, whether his condition is stable or deteriorating, and what this means to him and his family in terms of everyday activities (i.e. dressing, crossing streets, reading, going to school, holding a job, taking care of the house).

If the social workers sense a lack of knowledge, fear, or confusion about the eye diagnosis from either the patient or his family, we ask the clinic doctor to discuss with the patient and often with the family the eye disease and what it might mean in terms of limiting or not limiting his activities. Often we ask the referring ophthalmologist to further clarify for the patient the diagnosis or particular treatment. Ongoing communication between the referring ophthalmologist and our clinic staff is essential. In order for the patient to assume responsibility for his own rehabilitation, i.e. be the leader of his team, he must at least understand his diagnosis.

The social worker must know the patient's financial resources to determine how professional services and devices will be paid. We are careful to use all possible third parties and special private funds whenever possible. No patient is refused service for lack of funds. The social worker also helps the patient with any transportation problems.

Knowledge of living arrangements can be important in determining what type of device might be effective and whether family members can be counted on to help or hinder a patient's struggle for greater independence. Parents or spouses often need considerable help in allowing the patient the freedom to grow independent through exploration of numerous, previously untried activities.

The patient may be depressed. This depression is often a normal reaction to loss of sight, and the social worker helps the patient and his family develop the confidence needed to live through this depression and go on to rebuild a meaningful life. If the patient is thought to be suicidal or severely emotionally disturbed, psychiatric help is sought. Psychiatric help is always available from our psychiatric consultant.

The social worker coordinates additional services provided by other agencies or professionals so that minimal duplication, confusion, or gaps occur. Each patient is encouraged to take an active and responsible role in his own rehabilitation. This requires the patient to have a thorough knowledge of his visual diagnosis and prognosis and the options available to him so that he can meaningfully reject or accept what the staff is offering him. Effort is made to ensure the patients of realistic expectations of what other agencies or professionals can provide.

Follow-up care is monitored by the social worker, and patients are instructed to return yearly or whenever additional problems occur. Social workers maintain follow-up files; and, when we do not hear from a patient or he misses an appointment, we offer additional appointments and try to resolve any difficulties about coming to the Clinic.

Social Work Student Teaching

Two graduate students in social work from the Boston University School of Social Work do their first year fieldwork training for a period of seven months in our clinic. They carry a limited case load and are supervised by the clinic staff social workers. These students present cases at our staff meetings in conjunction with clinic doctors and the consulting psychiatrist. They also make home visits to patients.

Our staff and our students are encouraged to examine their own feelings and attitudes towards blindness, serious illness, and death. Each professional must understand his own feelings and prejudices if he is to establish an effective therapeutic climate for his patients.

Group Counseling

Group counseling is beginning to develop in our clinic. Our group, at present, consists of middle-aged persons. It is felt that there are a great many frustrations and issues that our patients and their families need to discuss. It is often difficult for them to find other people with similar problems with whom they can discuss these problems. Group sessions provide an opportunity to explore feelings and attitudes. Our group is selected and led by a clinical psychologist and a social worker. We plan additional groups.

Summary

The Vision Rehabilitation Clinic social workers, along with the clinic doctors, referring ophthalmologists, and pertinent community agencies help each patient to direct his efforts towards greater personal independence and maximum utilization of his remaining vision.

THE ROLE OF THE OPTOMETRIST

John E. Asarkof

Introduction

The Vision Rehabilitation Clinic at Boston University Medical Center in Boston first commenced operation in the latter part of 1968 and received patients one afternoon per week. The staff consisted of an optometrist and an ophthalmologist.

From this beginning we have expanded to five clinic days per week. The staff presently consists of an ophthalmologist who functions as the medical director; three optometrists, one of whom is optometric director of the clinic and serves as the liaison between the clinic and the Massachusetts College of Optometry; one full-time social worker and two part-time social workers, one of whom serves as the administrative director of the clinic; and a full-time administrative assistant. In the past month an ophthalmic assistant who assists in training patients in the use of low vision devices and assists the ophthalmologist has been added to the staff.

The social workers' duties consist of interviewing the patient to discuss his needs and problems, either physical or emotional, and arranging for psychiatric consultation if indicated. They act as a liaison between the Commission for the Blind and the clinic in problems concerning payment for devices, payment for tuition in schools and colleges, and vocational rehabilitation.

The administrative assistant is in charge of records, reports on patients from all referring sources, and general secretarial work.

The optometrists examine patients, train patients in the use of low vision devices, and also design devices in special cases. They fit and adjust spectacles and place special emphasis on the fitting and adjusting of head born telescopes. The fitting of high-powered bifocals is much more critical than the fitting of conventional bifocals because of the much closer working distance which makes it necessary to fit the segments much higher than one would ordinarily. Because of this fact, the optometrists prefer either to fit these devices themselves or write specific instructions if a prescription is given to the patient. The visual needs or other problems that the patient may experience are discussed with the optometrist by the social worker following the interview with the patient.

Four senior optometric students from the Massachusetts College of Optometry rotate through the clinic for a three-month period. Prior to this rotation the students have had a series of lectures on the optics of low vision devices, the pathology of low vision, and the low vision examination. The students have also been exposed to routine refractions in the General Clinic of the Massachusetts College of Optometry for a period of 1½ years before commencing any clinical work in low vision. The students are supervised by members of the faculty of the College of Optometry at the General Clinic, and by the staff optometrist at the Vision Rehabilitation Clinic. Their activities at first consist of observing the optometrist and ophthalmologist examining patients. Later, as they become more skillful and adept at handling patients, they perform the examinations under optometric supervision.

The optometrist also participates in the design and development of new equipment; and we recently had constructed, with the cooperation and assistance of the American Optical Company, a rear projection, zoom lens acuity-measuring device. By means of remote controls, the letter size can be changed to measure acuities from 20/70 to 20/1000.

The *loan system,* or the system of loaning various devices to patients before a definitive device is prescribed, is used routinely for arriving at a prescription for patients. This system was adopted with modifications from the New York Lighthouse. We are all aware of the fact that examining the patient in a controlled clinical environment and then having the patient function adequately with a device in his place of employment, school, or home may create many problems. Telescopes for distance, head born reading glasses of all types, and hand and stand magnifiers are maintained in the clinic stock so that they are readily available for loan.

One or more devices may be loaned to a patient; and, when the patient returns to the clinic and the device appears to work out adequately, it is prescribed. If the low vision aid does not prove to be sufficient for the patient's needs, others are readily available for trial until the optimum prescription is arrived at. The loan system works particularly well for variable conditions such as diabetic retinopathy, in which the condition may vary from one month to the next.

One of the features of this program is the fact that the patients are seen by the same examiner on each visit until the completion of the case. This tends to give the patient a feeling that the doctor has a better understanding of his or her case and, indeed, does assist the examiner in determining what can be done to help the patient to the greatest extent.

Following the prescription of a device or devices, either of stock nature or made up to a specific prescription, and after the patient has used the device for six weeks, a follow-up appointment is made. At this time the patient is questioned as to how he is getting along and if there are any problems. Patients are then requested to return in one year unless there are problems prior to this time. Six months after using the device, a questionnaire printed in large type (24 point) is sent to the patient, an example of which appears in Figure XXIX-I.

An optometrist is in charge of ordering devices and of seeing that an adequate supply of loan devices is available at all times.

The ophthalmologist, optometrist, and social worker work together in full cooperation. If the patient has not had an ophthalmological

NAME:
ADDRESS:

TELEPHONE:
DOCTOR:

1. **WAS A LOW VISION DEVICE OR DEVICES PRESCRIBED FOR YOU?**

2. **WHAT WAS IT (MAGNIFIER, TELESCOPE, ETC.)**

3. **IF SO, ARE YOU STILL USING IT?**

4. **IS IT HELPFUL?**

5. **PLEASE LIST THE THINGS THAT YOU CAN DO WITH IT THAT YOU WERE UNABLE TO DO BEFORE.**

6. **ARE YOU EXPERIENCING ANY DIFFICULTY WITH YOUR LOW VISION DEVICE?**

7. **IF YES, PLEASE EXPLAIN (I.E. VISION WORSE, DEVICE BROKEN, HEALTH PROBLEM, LIGHTING INADEQUATE, ETC.)**

Figure XXIX-1. A follow-up questionnaire in 24-point type sent to low vision patients six months after the initial visit.

evaluation within six months prior to being seen at the clinic, the staff ophthalmologist takes care of this part of the evaluation.

Monthly staff meetings are held at which time administrative and other problems concerning the adequate functioning of the clinic are discussed. Case presentations are given by the optometric students, the ophthalmology resident who rotates through the clinic, and the graduate social work students who do their work in the clinic. A psychiatry resident is present at the staff meetings and assists in counseling and attempting to solve many problems which the low vision patient might have.

Lectures to staffs of organizations which care for the blind or partially sighted are given by the ophthalmologist, the optometrists, or social workers who staff the clinic. Talks to lay organizations and film presentations of *LOW VISION: The Edge of Sight** are given for informative as well as fund-raising activities.

We have learned a great deal about the handling of the partially sighted since 1968, and we are now more than ever convinced of the necessity of the team approach in adequately caring for these patients. The social worker, vocational rehabilitation counselor, peripatologist, psychiatrist, ophthalmologist, and optometrist must all work together and be involved in attempting to solve the many and varied problems of the low vision patient.

---

* *LOW VISION: The Edge of Sight* is a thirty minute, sixteen millimeter color film in which four patients tell of their problems with low vision and show how they are resolving their visual difficulties through help from the Vision Rehabilitation Clinic at the Boston University Medical Center.

· CHAPTER XXX ·

The Low Vision Clinic: University of Alabama School of Optometry

THE ROLE OF THE LOW VISION TECHNICIAN

Randall T. Jose
and LoRetta McAdams

Introduction

THE PURPOSE of this presentation will be to propose the development of a formally structured educational program in low vision services for the optometric assistant. The proposed curriculum will be based on the Optometric Technician's Program as it is presently being offered at the School of Optometry, the Medical Center, University of Alabama in Birmingham with specialized training provided in the school's low vision clinic.

Patients are referred to the clinic from the vocational training program at the Alabama Institute for the Deaf and Blind, the Alabama School for the Blind, the Helen Keller School for the Deaf-Blind, Alabama Industries for the Blind, special education resource facilities, and private referrals from rehabilitation counselors, teachers, local optometrists, and ophthalmologists.

The low vision clinic is available to the public two days a week. The fourth year optometry interns and student optometric technicians work with patients under the supervision of a faculty instructor, our staff optometric (low vision) technician, and our staff social worker. This is a teaching institution, so no professional service fees are charged. A moderate registration fee for administrative costs is required. Optical aids are provided at cost plus a modest prescription service fee. Indigent care is provided through our social worker when needed.

The patient spends approximately two hours at each of the first two visits. At the end of this four to five-hour evaluation, it is hoped that a permanent aid can be prescribed and a training program initiated. The involvement of the family, teachers, and counselors in the examination is encouraged. The student is expected to involve himself with as many outside professionals as possible within the structure of the clinical program.

Model Examination

The examination procedure which is used as our model service for the clinic is described below.

1. Appointment: the patient is identified as a low vision patient. Objective data are obtained such as patient's name, address, age, phone, spouse/parent, and referral sources. If the patient has been referred, a request is sent to the referring doctor or agency for all available data and opinions. It is then determined if only an evaluation is required or if complete services are to be rendered. This sequence of service can be provided by a receptionist, secretary, or administrator.

2. Initial Introduction: as the patient arrives for the appointment, a brief introduction to the services is provided. The examination procedure is explained and an orientation to optical aids provided. Realistic expectations about the impending examination and the procedures that follow are developed. This time should also be used by the doctor to introduce the technician as one of the team members. This can be handled by the doctor in conjunction with the low vision technician, orthoptist, nurse familiar with low vision care, or other such experienced staff.

3. Case History: the case history is taken in order to obtain *subjective* diagnostic data to familiarize the examiner with the patient's needs and to direct the examiner's attention towards areas stressed in the diagnostic evaluation to follow. This service can be handled by the doctor, low vision technician, the social worker, or nurse. (See Appendix A.)

4. Diagnostic Evaluation: diagnostic data are collected by both the technician and examiner. The technician can obtain information about visual acuities, keratometry, visual fields, tonometry, color vision, binocularity, and eccentric viewing. The doctor

may wish to collect these data or the technician may perform these services while the doctor attends to other patient responsibilities. Although acuities and visual field screening tests are often performed in offices today by staff members, a much better evaluation of these pertinent tests can be provided by technicians due to their more extensive educational background. They are more familiar with the principles behind each test and of factors affecting its results.

5. Neutralization of Present Prescriptions: while the examiner reviews the history and data collected by the technician and expands upon the initial case history, neutralization of all the patient's present prescriptions and identification of all optical aids presently being used by the patient may be performed. This service can be provided by the low vision technician or staff optician if available.

6. Tentative Prescription: the doctor now performs a series of tests to determine the presence of any significant refractive error, i.e. retinoscopy, trial frame subjective, telescopic subjective. Near-point performance is evaluated; then, based upon these results and the data already collected, a tentative treatment program is determined. This program is discussed with the patient. The tentative aid is loaned to the patient for training. Most practitioners will agree that this is the responsibility of the doctor. The proposed program will not provide training in these areas for the technician.

7. Demonstration of Optical and Nonoptical Aids: the technician again explains to the patient the proposed treatment program. The use of the tentative prescription is demonstrated and a training program is developed. The patient is trained to use the aid and must demonstrate a certain proficiency with the aid before it is loaned for home use. At this time the patient is introduced to a variety of nonoptical aids. This will give the patient the time prior to the next visit to consider applications of these aids at home. This training service is rarely performed by the examiner due to time limitations, so the technician can well serve the patient in this capacity. This service can also be provided by a nurse or some other low vision staff specialist who is familiar

with the advantages and disadvantages of optical and nonoptical aids and understands the optical service being offered the patient.

8. Dispensing: at the end of the first visit either the *loaner* aid is dispensed to the patient and/or measurement and frame selection are taken for a permanent optical aid or conventional correction. The technician or optician can perform this service. The doctor will usually serve in a supervisory capacity.

9. Posthistory: after the completion of the first examination, the patient is referred for an interview with a social worker *trained in the area of low vision care*. The history should be specifically geared to the low vision service and include data on patient expectations, motivations, family situations, family history, and also a general description of the patient's attitudes towards his vision loss. Most important, the social worker finds out if the examination and proposed treatment program seem to be meeting the patient's needs as stated and if they are in keeping with his expectations. The social worker discovers if the patient feels that the examiner and staff understood his needs and if the patient is benefiting from the service. As a result of this history and the diagnostic data, the social worker may recognize a need for additional services for the patient: a psychological evaluation to determine mental abilities, visual auditory memory, or fine coordination; a report from an educator or counselor about the educational or vocational progress of the patient; or a request for more intensive therapy or casework. An interview with the family by the social worker may be of benefit. When possible, immediate family or those living with the patient should be contacted and told about the treatment program. In this way they can serve to reinforce the patient's desires to function visually. A sample history is found in Appendix B. The social worker is hard to replace in the rendering of this service. A less comprehensive posthistory can be administered by the technician, nurse, or low vision specialist, but this defeats the purpose of a third noninvolved party evaluating the success of the diagnostic procedures.

10. If the social worker senses any problems related to the aid, the

technician reviews the home-training program with the patient and the aid. The technician tries to insure that the patient has the correct aid and will not become frustrated and consequently fail to return for follow-up visits. Upon completion of the interview, the social worker may wish to review the case with the staff.

11. Progress History: a progress history is taken at the time of the second appointment. This information is taken to determine the patient's success in using the aid at home, problems encountered in its use, and, in general, the patient's confidence in using his residual vision. Materials with which the patient works are brought in for this examination. The doctor, low vision technician, nurse, or low vision staff specialists can all provide this service.

12. Second Visit: the examiner now has the diagnostic data as well as a comprehensive history compiled from the first visit. The patient has been involved in a training program and has been using the aid for several weeks to determine for himself what difficulties are experienced with the aid. The second visit is scheduled to evaluate the patient's progress and problems with the loaner device and allows for further testing to determine a final prescription. The second examination has as its primary objective the coordination of all data collected into a final prescription. All this information is used by the examiner to determine the prescription(s) that will provide the patient with maximum utilization of his residual vision. The patient must be reassured that he can function visually. This procedure is the responsibility of the doctor. Depending on the type of evaluation conducted, the low vision technician will probably provide a great deal of chairside assistance during this period.

Depending on the proficiency of the patient in using his aid, a number of training sessions may have to be scheduled. These sessions reinforce the patient's use of the aid and also allow him the opportunity to express his problems in using the aid. The low vision technician provides this training service. Having participated in the determination of the prescription, the technician can easily evaluate the patient's progress with the aid.

Major problems can be brought immediately to the attention of the doctor.
13. Examination Summary and Reports: a low vision clinic functions as a consultation service. Summaries of findings in a comprehensive report are an essential part of any referral service. Pertinent data should be brief and meaningful. Performance of the patient should be noted. Recommendations for the prescription and other services should be clearly defined. (Appendix C shows two sample forms, the Birmingham Clinic and the New York Lighthouse Clinic.)
14. Follow-up Care: the revisit appointment is scheduled depending upon the individual case. Patients with stable eye conditions may be seen according to need, perhaps in two years or more. Patients with an unpredictable prognosis may be told to report at stated intervals, three to six months or when vision changes. Patients should feel free to request appointments if their visual needs change or if, for some reason, they fail to use their aid correctly. The revisit is the major responsibility of the doctor and the technician, but both must see the patient. The patient may need the services of the social worker even more at this visit, especially if there has been a deterioration of function.

The entire sequence of tests and evaluations presented might be considered a very comprehensive low vision examination. The total service cannot always be rendered, nor is such an extensive evaluation always desirable. However, the sequence does point out the total service that should be made available to those patients who can benefit from it.

APPENDIX A: LOW VISION FORMS

Case History

PATIENT OBJECTIVES:
1. Are you familiar with optical aids?
2. Do you think you can be helped by optical aids?
3. Do you use any aids now?
4. Are you satisfied with these aids?
5. Patient prefers: OD   OS.

VISUAL HISTORY:
1. When did you last have an eye examination?
2. Who was your doctor?
3. Treatment/surgery.
4. What have doctors told you caused your loss of vision?
5. Have you ever had a low vision examination?
6. Who was your doctor?
7. Recent changes.
8. Onset of loss.

MEDICAL HISTORY:
1. Last physical.
2. Doctor.
3. How did he say your health was at that time?
4. Your opinion of your health.
5. Medications.
6. Are you a diabetic? Treatment—

FAMILY HISTORY:
1. Does anyone in your family have the same eye condition?
2. Visual: Glaucoma, cataract, squint, other eye diseases?
3. Medical: Diabetes, hypertension.

MOBILITY:
1. Do you get around alone outdoors, even in strange places?
2. Do you use any mobility aids like a cane or a dog?
3. Do you have any difficulty in getting around indoors, even in strange places?
4. Observations.

DISTANCE VISION:
1. Able to see: billboards, labels———inches, faces at———ft.
2. Do you attend movies?
3. How close do you sit?
4. Do you watch TV?
5. Size screen———black/white or color.
6. Do you have any problem recognizing colors?

ILLUMINATION:
1. Do you see better and are your eyes more comfortable when it is bright and sunny or overcast and cloudy?

2. Do you use sunglasses?
3. Do you use a visor (hat)?
4. Are you bothered by glare when indoors? Some———Little ———None———.
5. Do you have more trouble with your vision at night than you do during the day?

NEAR VISION:
1. a. Do you read print?
   b. Can you read:

	Work Distance	Optical Aid/Rx
(1) Newspaper Headlines	———	———
(2) Large Print	———	———
(3) Textbooks	———	———
(4) Typed Print	———	———
(5) Magazines	———	———
(6) Newspaper	———	———
(7) Telephone Book	———	———
(8) Mail	———	———
(9) Bible	———	———

   c. How much reading do you do now?
   d. Which type print do you use most?
   e. What kind of light do you use for reading?
   f. Did you read more prior to your vision loss?
   g. How do you keep up with current news, etc.?
2. a. Do you use braille?
   b. Reader?
   c. Talking book or cassettes?

MOTIVATIONS:
1. Does patient:

   Sew   Have trouble with telephone
   Crochet   Write own checks
   Play cards   Write own correspondence
   Play musical instrument Do woodwork/household maintenance
   ———————
   Swim
   Bowl
   Bicycle ride
   Other activities

2. How do you spend your day?
3. Major activities.
4. If we can improve your vision with optical aids, are there any special tasks you would like us to concentrate on?
(Special problems?)

APPENDIX B: LOW VISION FORMS

Outline of Interview for Social Work Evaluation

I. Interview Summary:
   A. Background Information.
      1. Place of interview, time and date.
      2. Number of interviews.
      3. Persons involved in interview.
      4. Referral source and reason for referral.
      5. How much of the examination has previously taken place.
      6. What has been recommended so far.
      7. How patient feels about these recommendations and what he expects from them.

II. Patient-Personal Information:
   A. Physical Appearance.
   B. Attitude:
      1. Towards self and handicap.
      2. Towards others (family, friends, etc.).
      3. Towards social worker, doctor, etc..
   C. Interpretation of Visual Impairment and Medical Background Relating to It.
   D. Educational and/or Work History.
      1. Professional and/or vocational training.
      2. Previous positions held, degree of responsibility, length of time, salary, etc..
      3. Attitude toward:
         (a) Previous work history.
         (b) Towards own present abilities and future goals.
   E. Interests and Hobbies.
   F. Relationships, Family, Siblings, and Friends.
   G. Other Significant Factors.

III. Family Group:
   A. Members, Ages, Relationships.
   B. Parents or Parent Figures (for Children).
      1. Description.
      2. Personalities.
      3. Attitude towards client and handicap.
      4. Attitude towards agency and worker.
      5. Any significant cultural and/or religious factors.
   C. Marital History (for Adults) and Description of Other Significant Factors.

IV. Financial Situation.

V. Other Agency Contacts as Related by Client and/or Family.

VI. Workers Impressions.

VII. Plan.

The Low Vision Clinic

APPENDIX C: LOW VISION REPORT FORMS

Birmingham Clinic

---

the University of Alabama in Birmingham / UNIVERSITY STATION / BIRMINGHAM, ALABAMA 35294
the Medical Center / SCHOOL OF OPTOMETRY / LOW VISION CLINIC
EXAMINATION SUMMARY

TO: RE:

Conventional distance correction-acuity   Near Correction-acuity/test distance
RE_____   _____
LE_____   _____

UNAIDED DISTANT ACUITY   UNAIDED NEAR ACUITY/test distance   VISUAL FIELDS
RE_____ _____   _____
LE_____ _____   _____

COLOR VISION_____   HEALTH_____
RECOMMENDATIONS:
patient's needs:

exam findings:

aid recommended:

vocational/educational
enhancement from the aid:

Attention Instructors,
training required:

REHABILITATION PLAN REQUESTED:
  Optical Aid (s) _____
  Rx Service   _____   Janice Cummings, Social Worker
  Total Fee: _____   Randall T. Jose, O.D., Director Clinic for
                                      the Partially Sighted

APPENDIX C: LOW VISION REPORT FORMS

New York Lighthouse Clinic

FORM 4-24M-

The LIGHTHOUSE
THE NEW YORK ASSOCIATION FOR THE BLIND, INC.
111 EAST 59 STREET   NEW YORK, N.Y. 10022   TEL.: 355-2200

Date_____

To:

Re: was examined at the Low Vision Clinic
on   by   , M.D.

READING VISION			Diagnosis:
GAME		6 M	
CRANE		3.5 M	Best Distance Vision:
TOLD	26 (18 Pt)	2 M	sc OD cc OD
LEFT	387	1.6 M J10	OS OS
DOT	49 (12 Pt)	1.4 M	
BAKE	28 (9 Pt)	1 M J6	Reading Vision:
CODE	83	.8 M	
BOTH	84 (6 Pt)	.7 M	
	(4 Pt)	.5 M J1	
		.35 M	

18 Point Large Type Grades 1 - 3
14 Point Average Book Print Grades 4 - 7
12 Point Magazines, Books Grades 8 - 12
9 Point Magazines, Paper Back Books, Typing
7 Point Newspaper

SUMMARY

_____
Low Vision Service
N.Y. Assoc. for the Blind

LH001-(Rev. 3/73)

· CHAPTER XXXI ·

The Lighthouse Low Vision Service (New York)

THE OPHTHALMOLOGIST IN PATIENT MANAGEMENT

Eleanor E. Faye
and Clare M. Hood

Stage I: The Doctor

OPHTHALMOLOGISTS AND optometrists are trained to take from patients a detailed history related directly to the eye examination, or, let us say, to the reading process itself. Clinics have evolved detailed checklists and history sheets in an attempt to uncover all of the clues in a patient's life *before* he is examined.

We have assumed in the past that the history and diagnosis were the principle indicators of the correct prescription and the successful use of aids.

The traditional medical format of taking a history prior to or at the time of the patient's initial visit is not enough for the low vision patient.

Increasing the detail in the history, using checklists and complex forms does not reduce the failure rate or get at the individual who fails. Where does failure occur, and how can it be minimized?

One of the first things to recognize is that a detailed preliminary history may only tire the patient and distract the doctor with a mass of detail. Next, the follow-up should not occur too long after the initial examination when a patient is given a prescription to be filled and asked to return after he has received and used his glasses. If the prescription takes weeks to be filled, the follow-up visit is often delayed for weeks. We lose momentum with the patient and often lose the patient literally. A bad feature of delayed follow-up is that many average patients become disappointed and discouraged without supportive care: they project their negative reaction on the examiner and the aid. In other words, they fail.

If there is a gap between the initial visit and the follow-up, the borderline patient is too much on his own and without adequate information, energy, or perseverence to work with his aids once he has obtained them. A constructive step towards reducing this gap is to establish a loan system for glasses and some aids. The loan system is used only when the patient is not sure he wants glasses or when acceptance is in *d*oubt.

Immediately after the doctor's examination, the assistant takes the patient into the instruction room in which there is a complete selection of optical and nonoptical aids, work tables, and various lamps. The assistant then starts an intensive explanation and trial of the prescribed lenses. Patients at this time may reject the prescribed aid and start asking about other aids they see in the room. This information is taken back to the doctor and the suggested R_x is revised. There need be no confusion in the roles of the doctor and assistant if several facts are recognized.

First, medical and social *facts*, instead of being of prime importance, are only a preliminary to the major work of the low vision clinic. The greatest amount of time should be spent on teaching the patient to understand what he can do with his vision, to learn how aids work, and to apply what he has learned to what he wants to do.

Second, the assistant is in the ideal position to establish the type of relationship with the patient which will eventually allow the patient to put things together for himself. The relationship is similar to that of a teacher and pupil.

Third, it is necessary to have an intermediate stage in the low vision examination. This second phase, now called the instruction period, occurs immediately after the doctor's examination and precedes the follow-up.

The experience in the low vision clinic is a continuous education course for the patient *and* the staff member from the first visit through the follow-up. If the education process is valid and working properly, the patient will succeed, providing he is visually, physically, and emotionally capable.

The low vision examination falls naturally into three phases: the doctor's examination, the instruction period, and the follow-up.

Stage I: The Doctor's Examination of the Novice Patient

The patient is ignorant of what is expected of him, and, yet, he has unrealized expectations of what can be done for him. He needs reassurance that he can use his vision. He may be afraid of all the unknowns that have surrounded him since his vision was damaged.

The doctor fills an important function for the patient by determining the residual vision, confirming the diagnosis, and beginning to relate the remaining functional vision to the patient's needs. The examiner at this point can estimate the strength of aids which would be appropriate; but, other than testing the reading ability, he can only offer suggestions for aids.

In a clinic structure, the doctor has a clearly defined role which is backed up by the clinical assistant who has an equally well defined role. The doctor is no longer expected to make the perfect or final Rx.

It is his function to correlate the vision and the potential visual function, to interpret the fields and the influence of the pathology, and to make only a tentative prescription of aids and suggest to the assistant possibilities which might benefit the patient. He also reassures the patients medically. His history should be concerned with the medical and ophthalmological facts that are his responsibility in case management.

With this positive approach, the patient is not given time to go home and brood over his problems. He goes from the reassuring atmosphere of the eye examination to the second or instruction phase at which a peer takes over.

We have come to realize that the low vision experience is part of a continuous process that starts with the doctor's visit, is continued by a trained assistant, and ends with the follow-up.

THE LOW VISION ASSISTANT IN PATIENT MANAGEMENT

Stage II: The Assistant

In the instructional phase the patient has to begin to learn what low vision aids are and to relate aids to his own interest. The skilled assistant complements the initial history with a deeper probe into the patient's real reasons for the use of the aids. The instruction stage encompasses the nonintellectual pursuits of the patient, his daily needs, his reading habits, and begins to approach vocational possibilities.

Following the doctor's examination the low vision assistant takes the patient into a separate room. Family and friends should be included as part of the process.

The instruction room must be quiet and offer a certain degree of privacy. It should be fully equipped for instruction and follow-up.

Instruction Room

Hand Magnifiers	Nonoptical Aids
Stand Magnifiers	Printed Materials
Head Borne Aids	Large and Regular Type
Telescopes	Foreign Language Material
Closed Circuit TV	Writing Pads
Lamps of Several Varieties	Porous-tipped Pens

What does the assistant do?

1. Interprets the doctor's recommendations and clarifies misunderstandings (what the patient did *not* hear) that may have occurred during the initial examination.
2. Translates the doctor's tentative prescription and suggestions into the actual aids or combination of aids and shows the patient the range of aids and allows him to handle them in various combinations. The patient's reactions are observed.
3. Interprets his questions about the aids and instructs him in their proper use.
4. Improvises with different lens combinations if the patient does not seem to be responding to what is suggested.
5. Reports to the doctor any marked deviation in patient reaction.

The assistant relates as a peer. We all know from clinical experience that patients tend to show off for the doctor. They tell him what they think *he* wants to hear. They are afraid to touch on what they consider to be trivial or personal matters in the formal examination. With the assistant they feel more comfortable. During the instructional period the assistant is constantly aware of the patient's reaction and objectively evaluating the patient's mental attitude, his interest, his attention span, and his physical ability to use the aid. Members of the family also participate in the instruction, especially since they are to reinforce the instruction during the home-training period. When it seems appropriate, the assistant can suggest and interpret nonoptical aids to the patient. Patients usually inquire about cost. All aids in the instruction room are plainly marked, and the price list is posted. The final prescription is written when the doctor and assistant agree that the patient is ready.

Stage III: The Follow-up

The third stage of the examination is the follow-up and should follow within approximately two weeks. The staff now knows about the patient's real motives. The patient has a feeling of confidence in what he can do. Not only have his opinions and feelings been recognized, he has been allowed a choice.

Failure

Failure is a complex subject. When a case is to be terminated as a failure, it is not enough to write failure off by saying, "He lacks motivation," or "The patient is poorly motivated," or "The patient has to be motivated." All patients are "motivated;" that is, they want to *see*, but they may not be able to accept the amount of work it takes to learn to use their vision again in new ways.

If we have to say that our patient is not motivated, we are not stating the patient's case. Instead of talking about motivation, we put the case in the actual terms which describe the patient: the patient is depressed, the patient is mentally ill, the patient is retarded, he is reacting to his catastrophic blindness, or he has severe emotional problems. Put in realistic terms like this, we do not have to blame "motivation," a cliche which does not belong in a medical situation because it tells us nothing about the patient.

Failure for the low vision patient may not be the fault of the patient. He may not have the mental or physical ability to follow through or to accept the limitations of what is offered. It may also be the failure of the staff to recognize the patient's basic problems which might be other than visual.

Summary

In summary, the visual aid alone does not constitute rehabilitation.

Total management is a complex interaction of skilled history taking, expert medical attention, proper instructions; of sensitive social work; of appropriate referrals. All of this should add up to a realistic program of help for the patient.

SETTING UP A LOAN SYSTEM FOR OPTICAL AIDS

The Trial Program

In the examination procedure for the low vision patient, one of the most difficult areas for both the examiner and the patient is the selection of the final aid. It is not the calculation of the correct dioptric *strength* of the reading add for any given task that is difficult. The problem lies in a less concrete area which is based on experience rather than data. Because this is a new experience for the patient, he cannot know in advance what his visual impairment requires in the type of visual aid he uses. In order to relate low vision aids to daily existence, a patient must be able to try lenses in lifelike situations and to learn by doing.

In 1969 when statistics were analyzed from the Lighthouse Low Vision Clinic for the first six thousand patients (1953 to 1968), the success rate was found to be 64 percent, a figure which seemed low.[1] The clinic procedure was reviewed, and two areas of weakness emerged to explain this rather undistinguished record: the follow-up interval was often prolonged, and there was a long wait for a low vision prescription to be filled. The follow-up has been previously discussed. The solving of the prescription problem became known as the *loan system*, a lending library of spectacles, hand magnifiers, and telescopic devices.

The immediate effect of being able to give borderline patients a trial glass at their first visit was to remove the pressure from the staff of *having* to prescribe the correct lens at this visit. The long-term effect has been an increased success rate, from 64 percent to 81 percent success.

There is a logical reason for a *loan system* to be incorporated into every low vision clinic's structure. A patient is exposed to so many new ideas and stimuli that he can not be expected to sort out all this information at the first visit. The pressure of expectations for his performance loses momentum if he is simply sent out with a prescription and told to return when he gets his glasses. A surprising number of low vision patients need a definite schedule for a return visit for back-up training and reassurance and for counseling. If lenses can be offered on a true trial basis with no economic strings attached and no obligations other than participation in an evaluation, the patient's own decisions become important, and he can concentrate on his own experience and proceed at his own rate.

The Lighthouse Low Vision Clinic now gives 56 percent of its patients lenses on a trial basis, and these include spectacles, hand magnifiers, and telescopic devices.

When the loan system began, the trial period was a month. This led to administrative problems with too many lenses in circulation, a loss of patient interest, and a lag in staff-patient rapport. Reducing the trial period to three weeks increased the administrative chaos because of scheduling this awkward interval. The patient was still not getting enough reinforcement during the most critical period of his adjustment. The current two-week revisit schedule is ideal in terms of ease in scheduling and maintaining the patient's relationship with the assistant at a high energy level.

Case Histories

Case 1:

R.W., a sixty-three-year-old salesman with macular degeneration, was considering early retirement because he could no longer read the printouts or price sheets sent out by the companies he dealt with. He also could not manage his own orderbooks. To evaluate the printed material on the job, he took a +12 spectacle for the os, a +12 COIL hand magnifier, and a 3x illuminated pocket magnifier. In two weeks he rejected the spectacle because it overmagnified the computer numbers into a diffuse, blurred figure. He also rejected the 3x illuminated magnifier as a useless gadget. He immediately accepted and used the +12 COIL for brief spotting tasks. On reevaluation, the +8 with 10△ base-in provided just enough magnification for the print-outs, was cosmetically acceptable on the job, and he felt more comfortable using both eyes although there was a marked discrepancy in vision. Two weeks after the final prescription, he called back to order the 3x illuminated magnifier and stated that he had found a use for it; finding telephone numbers in poorly lit public telephone booths.

Case 2:

R.G., a seventy-two-year-old female, stated that her main interest was reading. She was given a 10x Keeler telemicroscope with a 5△ base-down prism (Press-On) applied to the ocular to allow reading with a comfortable head position. She needed a great deal of support which, in her case, meant weekly visits for counseling and training. It took four weeks for her to develop proficiency with the lens. After six weeks she realized that she really did not want to read that much and that she could not write with the 10x. She had the courage to request a lens for writing. A 5x Keeler telemicroscope allowed her to write and read back what she had written. This was given to her to try at home. She was relieved by not having to make the effort to read anymore. Here, a potential nonuser (or failure) was uncovered only after many weeks of supportive training. An expensive mistake was avoided, and the patient received the counseling which made the aid a success.

In these typical cases, the patients learned from experience based on actual use of the lenses.

Setting Up A *Loan* System

A system of lending optical devices has been in operation since 1969 at the Lighthouse Low Vision Clinic. The rest of this chapter will describe the operation of the current program.

Equipment

1. Frames. The least expensive, most efficient system is one which buys frames and stocks lenses from one optical company so that lenses and frames are interchangeable. As a rule, 44/22, 5¾ temple, P-3 (round) shape is easy to obtain.[2]
2. Monocular lenses with plano balance. If spectacles are made up with the reading lens in one eye only, more corrective lenses can be in circulation. After initial experience with frames made up with binocular corrections, the Lighthouse Clinic converted to monocular glasses.
3. Binocular lenses with clip-on occluders. Smaller clinics may find that binocular corrections cost less for the initial outlay and will reduce the size of the inventory.
4. Strength of lens engraved on temple. If stock lenses are supplied, they *must* be labeled in some permanent fashion to avoid

confusion. The optical company will do the engraving for a small fee. If the clinic prefers to make up loan lenses individually, the strength of the correction may be scratched into the lens carrier or corner of the lens.
5. Plastic bags. Lenses must be stored in disposable plastic bags to conform to department of health regulations.
6. Frame warmer. American Optical Company and Bausch and Lomb make an electric frame warmer.
7. Assortment of optical screwdrivers, screws, and pliers.
8. Dymo machine. Not recommended because the labels fall off after repeated washing.
9. Plastic occluders with foam padding.

Lens Inventory

The Lighthouse Low Vision Clinic uses American Optical AOlite® lenses[2] in the strengths outlined in Table XXXI-I. The lenses are listed in order of decreasing frequency of use.

When lenses were first given out on trial, the policy was not to lend small, inexpensive items such as hand magnifiers. However, the staff in charge of training soon found that hand and stand magnifiers were often needed as training devices and for use when the final prescription was divided between the spectacle add and a hand magnifier.[3] At present, higher strength magnifiers are in demand for training, especially to accustom a patient to the eventual prescription of a Designs for Vision, Type-R segment bifocal (which is not on loan). Magnifiers are listed in Table XXXI-II in order of decreasing frequency of use. At present, the only lens which we do not lend is the inexpensive Selsi +11. It was frequently not returned.

The loan system functions particularly well for telescopic devices. Their acceptance is not highly predictable. The 2.5x Selsi telescopes are loaned only to adults, not to children. The 2.2x wide angle Bioptic is often loaned to adults who need to experience telescopic distance vision firsthand. The 2.2x wide-angle lens is not given to patients for trial with driving because one patient took, and passed, his driver's test with it, and then did not buy it. If a patient who wishes to drive has made his decision and the telescope gives him the required acuity, he is given a direct prescription.

TABLE XXXI-I
SPECTACLES MOST COMMONLY LOANED
(IN DECREASING ORDER)

Dioptric Strength
+20
+24
+8 with 10△ base-in
+10 with 12△ base-in
+16
+12
+14
10x AO Microscopic
12x AO Microscopic
8x AO Microscopic
+6 with 8△ base-in

TABLE XXXI-II
MAGNIFIERS AND TELESCOPES MOST COMMONLY LOANED

Hand magnifiers	Telescopes
+20 COIL	6x-8x Selsi
+5 COIL (chest and hand magnifier)	2.5x Selsi
+12 COIL	2.8x Selsi
Jupiter 9 D	2.2x Wide-angle Bioptic (mounted in a frame)
+28 B&L (7x)	8x Zeiss
+32 B&L (10x)	
+7 COIL	
+17.6 COIL stand	
+5 Edroy	
+15 Sloan stand	
+4.7 Planoconvex	

Keeler wide-angle and binocular telemicroscopic systems work well in a loan inventory because they can be quickly exchanged in the trial frame and are simple to unscrew from the carriers. The initial outlay for stock lenses would be high, however, and delivery may be somewhat slow for final prescriptions. A large clinic would do well to work out arrangements directly with the American branch of the company.

Maintenance

After return, glasses are repaired, washed by immersion in soap and water, dried, and put in disposable plastic bags.

Storage

Lenses are stored in plastic bags inserted into a soft eyeglass case. They are kept in individual envelopes, filed in a filing cabinet by lens strength and corrected eye.

Life of Lenses

The average number of times a lens can be circulated before it is scratched or damaged is twenty-seven. Old lenses are retired as demonstration and teaching models at lectures or on display boards. The loss of loan lenses from the Lighthouse Clinic has been 1.2 percent of 642 devices loaned in 1973, including the +20 COIL, +20 and +24 spectacles, and the Selsi 6-8x telescope.

Records

When the lens is out on loan, the envelope containing the patient's name is filed by the month of the return appointment.

Cost of Average Setup

The cost of basic lenses for a small adequate inventory is between seven hundred to one thousand dollars, depending on the quantity of each dioptric strength needed for an individual clinic.

Summary

Not all patients need their lenses on a trial basis. Many choices of ready-made reading spectacles and hand magnifiers are available from local sources and from the Lighthouse Optical Aids Service. Thus, delays in obtaining prescriptions need not prolong the patient's waiting time. However, there are many borderline cases in which experience is needed before the patient can accept an aid or even know quite what is right for his needs. Patients like to try aids in the environment and under the conditions in which they will be using their glasses. Low vision patients should not have to pay for an aid until it is proven useful. For these reasons, all low vision clinics should try to incorporate such a system into their clinic structure.

REFERENCES

1. Faye, Eleanor E.: *The Low Vision Patient.* New York, Grune and Stratton, p. 186, 1970.
2. *Catalogue of Optical Aids,* 3rd ed. rev. New York, New York Lighthouse Low Vision Service, 1973.
3. Faye, Eleanor E.: Ibid. p. 53.

· SECTION NINE ·
Training Programs in Low Vision Clinics

· CHAPTER XXXII ·

Instruction of the Ophthalmology Resident: Massachusetts Eye and Ear Infirmary

JOEL KRAUT

Introduction

FROM READING the papers in this symposium, one realizes and understands the great importance of training those individuals who will care for patients with visual disabilities. The number of patients with low vision problems will increase greatly in the future. This is due to several factors. The majority of patients who have declining vision are in the older age category. This group will increase in size because of many of our medical advances. Accompanying this increase in life expectancy is an increase in literacy and increasing desire of elderly patients to remain integrated into our visually oriented society. Patients are unwilling to accept a loss of vision, and rightfully so.

As life expectancy increases, however, there will be a greater number of patients with degenerative eye problems and with certain diseases such as diabetes mellitus, hypertension, and atherosclerosis who will develop severe visual problems. Social agencies have already begun mobilization to help these patients who have visual disabilities. We, as ophthalmologists, must also begin to develop programs to care for these patients and enable them to be restored to a fuller and more productive life.

The Training Program at the Massachusetts Eye and Ear Infirmary

It is important for every ophthalmological residency training program to include instructions in the ophthalmic care of the patient with a low vision problem. These programs should include an understanding of the various disease states which contribute to creating a visual disability and an approach to those children and those adults who have impaired vision. As Dr. Seidenberg has pointed out, there are different approaches to children with these problems.[1] One must be able to perceive the proper questions to ask these patients. It is important to be able to test the vision and later follow through with the best recommendations. When dealing with children, it is important to understand and accurately assess each problem as well as the family's relationship and understanding of the visual disability.

I would like to describe the training program we have at the Massachusetts Eye and Ear Infirmary in Boston and some of our findings and impressions. Our low vision center is staffed with an ophthalmologist, an optometrist, ophthalmology residents, and ophthalmic technicians. The clinic serves as a center for clinic and privately referred patients with subnormal vision and also as a training center for our resident physicians in ophthalmology and our ophthalmic technicians.

Each ophthalmology resident is instructed in low vision in the basic science course and spends six weeks in the low vision center. These second-year resident physicians are carefully trained to evaluate each patient, reconfirm the past diagnosis, and understand the problem in relation to the particular patient. They then must perform an accurate low vision examination and recommend as to future disposition. This may involve prescribing a specific device or a nonoptical device. It may involve teaching the patient to properly utilize a device or spectacle that he or she already has but has not been using properly. It may be necessary and helpful to refer a patient to a public or private agency which may be of great assistance to a particular patient. We are fortunate in the Boston area to have many excellent public agencies and such privately endowed agencies as the Boston Aid to the Blind and the Carroll Rehabilitative Center, to name only two. It may involve explaining to the parents of a child the future expectations. We attempt to explain realistically to the parents of children with vision disability and to our adult patients what they can expect in the future. The physician performs all of these functions together in consultation with the staff members of our clinic.

The full-time staff optometrist is involved in performing the low vision evaluation and in instructing, along with the ophthalmologist, the ophthalmology residents and ophthalmic technicians. He also mechanically adjusts, when necessary, the various prescribed low vision devices to suit each patient in regard to the desired task. We are also attempting to develop new low vision devices, and the optometrist is actively involved in this process.

We also have a training program for ophthalmic technicians at our hospital. These physician's assistants are instructed to work in many areas of ophthalmology under the guidance of an ophthalmologist. These technicians spend one-half day each week for the entire year of their second year of training in the low vision center. A low vision examination can be very lengthy and time consuming. Well-trained ophthalmic technicians can perform some sections of these examinations, including the taking of the history and the testing of visual acuities with the various low vision devices. This will allow any ophthalmologist or clinic to evaluate and care for more patients with these problems. Ophthalmic technicians can be of great assistance in ophthalmology by providing better care in many areas.

It is important for all major population areas to have low vision centers to which patients can be referred for evaluation of visual disabilities. It is equally important, however, for each ophthalmologist in practice to understand how to perform a satisfactory low vision examination. In our training program, we attempt to teach this dual approach for several reasons.

The Low Vision Examination

First, as has been pointed out by Dr. Moore, many of the low vision prescriptions involve the use of the normal refractive techniques.[1] As long as one understands some of the basic laws of optics and instructs the patient carefully in the practical applications of these laws, it is not difficult for every ophthalmologist to perform a low vision examination. As Dr. Faye has explained, some of her most valuable low vision devices are high plus spectacle lenses.[1] If a patient is given one of these spectacles, it must be carefully explained that the material to be read must be held closer to the eyes in order to be visualized. Many of our elderly citizens had been told when they were youngsters that it was detrimental to the eyes to hold a book close to the face when reading. It is important to instruct these low vision patients that the only way they will be able to read is by holding the reading material close to the eyes. They should be instructed that this will not damage their eyes.

Second, it is important for all ophthalmologists to be able to perform a satisfactory low vision examination because many of these patients do live a long distance from a low vision center, and it is difficult for them to travel to have an examination. In our clinic we examine patients referred to us by ophthalmologists and optometrists all over New England and even other areas of the country. It is a hardship for many to travel these considerable distances. Many of these elderly patients would prefer to be cared for by their own family ophthalmologist who may have followed them for many years and who can provide for the patient excellent follow-up examinations.

In our training program, the first half of the examination involves an in-depth interview with the patient and his family about his visual problems. We have found this to be very important in understanding and assisting those patients referred to us.

We ask all of our patients, for example, what problem they have with their eyes. As you can imagine, most patients referred to a low vision clinic have been examined by many physicians before coming to us. We were surprised when we reviewed the records of some 328 consecutive patients examined in 1971 and 1972 and found that eighty-six patients of this group said they did not know what the problem was with their eyes or said that they were never told. This number represents 26 percent of the total number of patients. Twenty-two of this group who thought they knew what was wrong with their eyes were, in fact, incorrect in their conceptions.

There are probably several reasons why such a large percentage of these patients deny knowledge of his or her eye problem. Many of our patients are elderly, and some may have been told and forgotten due to cerebral vascular insufficiency. Some of these patients may not have been told about their ocular problems and may not have inquired. Father Carroll in his book *Blindness* described an individual's loss of vision as an act of dying.[2] Many of our patients deny to themselves, their families, and to us that their life must change and that things will never be as they once were. Part of our training program is to teach our staff how to help these patients to use the residual vision that they still have. We have found that unless we can do this, no low vision device will be helpful.

We train our residents and ophthalmic technicians to find out the reason each patient has come to the center and how we can best help him. In our clinic more than 70 percent of the patients are sixty years of age or older. The most common problem we encounter is macular pathology, mainly macular degeneration. Approximately 80 percent of all patients express as their primary goal the desire to be able to read again. This is a most reasonable and realistic goal, and every effort should be made to train every future ophthalmologist, optometrist, and ophthalmic technician to enable our patients to read again.

Program Coordination

In our hospital we attempt to coordinate our activities with those of the other departments in regard to patient care and research. In the Laboratory of Retinal Degenerations, Dr. Eliot L. Berson has been investigating the use of a night vision device as an aid for those patients with defective retinal rod function. These are patients with night blindness problems such as retinitis pigmentosa and stationary night blindness. The original or Generation I night vision device was originally devised for military use to be fitted over a rifle and is almost 3 pounds in weight and 14 inches long. This device allows one to see with minimal illumination, and one has to have only cone vision to see. It emits no radiation of its own but captures single photons on a photocathode which are then in turn converted into electrons which are accelerated through an electric field. These electrons then excite a P20 phospor screen enabling retinal cones to function and permitting vision. This bulky device has been modified into a second generation image intensifier device which is a pocketscope with a weight of 0.8 pounds and a length of 5 inches.

In our center, many other devices which are not as sophisticated as this night vision device are also being evaluated for use as possible low vision devices. Our residents, ophthalmic technicians, and staff are each involved in this clinical research.

Another aspect of our training program, aside from the examination and prescription of aids, is the resident's evaluation of the patient's success with his optical or nonoptical device. He also learns to refer the patient to another clinic or physician if he feels further treatment would be helpful, e.g. a patient with a retinal problem might benefit from laser treatment.

In summary I feel that it is important for all centers of ophthalmology to train their physicians in the techniques of assisting the adult or the child with partial vision.

REFERENCES

1. Faye, Eleanor E., and Hood, Clare M., et al.: *Low Vision*. Springfield, Thomas, 1975.
2. Carroll, Rev. T. J.: *Blindness*. Boston, Little, Brown, 1961.

CHAPTER XXXIII

A Resident's View of Low Vision Training

Gwen K. Sterns

Introduction

Low vision training should be considered an integral part of every ophthalmology resident's education. Traditional residency training programs place emphasis on the patient's disease and his medical and surgical management. Equal emphasis should be placed on the patient's visual function,[1] i.e. the degree of visual impairment produced by disease and the means available for dealing with that visual impairment.

Instruction in low vision varies from one residency program to another. Some residency training programs have weekly clinics for low vision patients under close supervision by trained personnel. Other programs have very little training in this field. In the New York metropolitan area, ophthalmology residents have the advantage of exposure to a major low vision center, the Lighthouse. The opportunity exists to meet and work with the Lighthouse personnel who give training in the management of low vision patients. Residents are able to gain familiarity with the low vision optical and nonoptical equipment, to observe the patients utilizing the available aids, and to participate in the prescribing of low vision aids under the supervision of a trained staff.

The experience at a low vision center is a valuable one. This experience however, must be reinforced in the resident's own program. Further, not every resident training program has the advantage of being close to a large low vision center. Therefore, other methods for training in the field of low vision must be incorporated into ophthalmology training programs.[2]

The following are suggestions for the incorporation of low vision training into ophthalmology residents' curriculum.

Low Vision Training in the Basic Science Course

Most ophthalmology residency training programs include a basic science course. Inclusion of training in low vision in this course would serve to keep the residents up to date as to the aids and services available. Those residents not previously exposed to low vision training would be given a good introduction to the techniques and aids available.

Establishment of Low Vision Clinics within the Residency Program

Low vision clinics could be run on a weekly, biweekly, or monthly basis depending on patient need. A trained supervisory staff of either ophthalmologists or optometrists should be available for instruction and consultation. The clinic should contain a trial set of low vision optical and nonoptical aids.[3]

Regional Conferences in the Field of Low Vision

Regional conferences would enable current ideas and techniques to be presented and an exchange of methods and technology to take place.

Literature and Films on Low Vision Aids

General availability of literature[4,5] and films[2,6] dealing with the types of aids available would keep residents and practitioners up to date on the available aids, the means of obtaining them, and their relative cost to the patient. Films could demonstrate the use of the aid, its value, and its limitations. This would be important for those residents in programs not located near a low vision center.

Training at Major Low Vision Centers

Residents should, when possible, be encouraged to observe and participate at established low vision centers.[7] This allows the resident to gain familiarity with current techniques and equipment as well as facilities available for the referral of problem patients in his region.

The incorporation of some or all of the above suggestions into the ophthalmology residency training program would enable more ophthalmologists to be trained in low vision and to develop an awareness of the problems and solutions unique to the low vision patient. The general ophthalmologist would then be competent to handle many uncomplicated low vision patients in his own practice and to use the low vision center for more comprehensive care of problem patients.

REFERENCES

1. American Foundation for the Blind: Not without sight. New York, 19½ min., 16mm color film, 1973.
2. Low vision patients. American Academy of Ophthalmology and Otolaryngology, 38 min. videotape, 1974.
3. *Catalogue of Optical Aids*, 3rd ed. rev. New York, New York Lighthouse Low Vision Service, 1973.
4. Faye, Eleanor E.: *The Low Vision Patient*. New York, Grune and Stratton, 1970.
5. Fonda, Gerald: *Management of the Patient With Subnormal Vision*, 2nd ed. St. Louis, Mosby, 1971.
6. New York Association for the Blind: The low vision patient. New York, 20 min., 16 mm color training film, 1970.
7. *Directory of Low Vision Aids Facilities in the United States*. New York, National Society for the Prevention of Blindness, Inc., 1973-1974.

· CHAPTER XXXIV ·

A Training Program for the Low Vision Technician

RANDALL T. JOSE

AT PRESENT, there are two basic types of paraprofessional training programs in the eye care field: the ophthalmic assistant who serves as an assistant to the ophthalmologist and the optometric technician who obviously works as a chairside assistant to the optometrist. I will not define the philosophies of each training program as they are still new and dynamic programs which will continue to reflect the changing attitudes of the respective professions they serve.[1,2]

We will be using as our standard of reference the optometric technician program. This is a matter of convenience, however, and is not to suggest that the ophthalmic assistants cannot function in the capacity of an assistant in the low vision examination.

Levels of Responsibility

Three levels of responsibility can be defined within paraprofessional training programs: the low vision assistant, the technician, and the technologist. Not all clinics require a low vision training program that reflects these three levels of training. The scope of duties performed by the proposed paraprofessionals will depend on the type of institution, clinic, or practice in which the services are to be rendered. For our purposes, we will define the responsibilities of a low vision technician. Other clinics may require further definition of the assistant and technologist.[3,4]

The term technician will be used throughout this paper, but it is not meant to serve as any limitation to the program. Many clinics refer to this person as the *assistant* as has been previously mentioned.

The low vision technician offers several advantages in the provision of vision care services to the partially sighted. Obviously, correct utilization of technicians in the various low vision centers will allow the clinic staff to be able to provide services for more people in this area.

The technician's skills and responsibility for patient care will give the practitioner more time to perform an evaluation of the patient and become involved in a rehabilitative rather than merely a diagnostic type of service. This is particularly important for large clinics in which a great number of people are being seen and time is at a premium. A significant increase in truly successful cases will be realized as a more rehabilitative emphasis is brought to the services presently being offered. *The technician can be the means for providing the extra training that can mean so much to a patient.* Not only will some failures be prevented, but the success cases can also be much more significant in rehabilitating a patient into a socially and economically acceptable life style.

The technician's interaction with other professional groups involved in the total rehabilitation program (social services, communication skills, mobility) will enhance the success of the optical aids program and will also contribute to the patient's participation in these other services.

A Training Program for the Low Vision Technician

No *one* training program can possibly reflect the examination techniques practiced by all of the doctors and clinics involved in low vision. Those aspects of this model which do not apply to a particular method of practice can either be disregarded or serve as food for thought as to how this service might be incorporated into present procedures.

The instructional material covered during the training program must be presented in such a manner that the technician will not graduate with an inflexible diagnostic procedure in working with low vision patients. The emphasis of the training will be on making the students comfortable and confident in working with the partially sighted, on giving the students enough exposure to the care of the partially sighted so as to give them a better understanding of the needs of this population, and on providing them with a comprehensive set of *basic* skills upon which they can build. To achieve these objectives, the technician's curriculum must include the following board areas of training.

1. General Diagnostic Procedures: principles of case history taking, basic pharmacology of eye medication (miotics, mydriatics, diuretics, and other commonly used drugs), dispensing techniques, visual fields, patient management, keratometry, visual acuity, and color vision.

The technician must fully develop these techniques in working with the routine low vision patient. This experience will serve as a basis for development and understanding the needs of the partially sighted patient both in the administration of the various examination tests and in the subsequent training procedures. Simply stated, the technician must be able to handle routine cases before tackling the more difficult ones.

2. Orientation to Low Vision: the technician will be given instruction in the special needs of the partially sighted and blind. Statistics on the prevalence and causes of blindness and visual loss will be presented. The psychological considerations in working with the partially sighted and a review of the availability of other professional services will be discussed. The student will be exposed to the blind and partially sighted in various educational, vocational, and social settings. The key word is exposure with *insight*.

The technician must be given the opportunity to interact with the partially sighted and blind. This exposure will help the technician be secure when working with them. To help them adjust to the uncomfortable feeling many people get when they first start working closely with "blind people," they need to develop a psychological insight into their own attitudes toward blindness.[5]

3. Introduction to the Low Vision Examination: specific tests will be reintroduced to the student. Special techniques or modifications of these routine procedures for administration to the partially sighted patient will be presented, i.e. acuities, visual fields, history. The technician will be introduced to the principles of magnification and made familiar with an inventory of diagnostic optical and nonoptical aids and their availability.

The technician will learn to modify previously learned standard techniques to the low vision evaluation. To insure the technician's success in working with optical aids, a lecture course will be given that discusses the principles of microscopic and telescopic magnification. Basic lens design will be reviewed. Verification of aids and dispensing techniques will also be presented at this time. A standardized list of optical and nonoptical aids will have to be developed so as to expose the technician to those aids used in most of the established clinics and practices. The list might appropriately reflect those aids in common use.

4. Training and Follow-Up Care: a combination of lecture presentations and clinical experiences will familiarize the technician with the utilization and limitations of optical aids. The technician will learn techniques to train patients to use their aids correctly and to recognize problem areas and methods used in handling these problems, i.e. when to refer back to the examiner. How to use the professional services of social workers, educators, and rehabilitation instructors will be stressed as part of the interdisciplinary approach.

The training aspect of low vision care is a common thread throughout all established and successful low vision clinical programs. It is in the area of training and follow-up care that the technician will probably most benefit any program. Some programs may use the technician *only* for these services. Even if so limited, the entire educational training program of the technician will be utilized, and an enjoyable and challenging career can still be realized. To enhance the technician's training, it is strongly suggested that the technician participate in some chairside activities. This increases the quality of the clinical training because the technician is involved with the diagnostic aspects of the evaluation. It gives the doctor-technician team the opportunity to share ideas and discuss interpretation of patient's expressed needs. This type of involvement in the total service allows the technician to understand the doctor's recommendations for the treatment program and effectively follow through.

Follow-up care is often neglected in working with the partially sighted. A specific model cannot be presented because the type of follow-up program will vary from one clinic situation to the next.

The importance of follow-up care will be stressed and the student will be exposed to the system established at the training program.

5. Internship: the initial training program cannot reflect all clinical attitudes and approaches to patient care. The internship will broaden the technicians' clinical experience and increase their flexibility through exposure to these different clinical situations.

The value of the internship will be to expose the student to a new set of treatment concepts. It will force the students to use their training background to make judgments regarding different approaches to care. If handled correctly this experience can contribute to the technician's skills and confidence in handling the responsibility of patient care. Such an experience will also give students a more concentrated exposure to patients.

The internship may even be completed at the future site of employment if that is known. More than likely it will occur in a predetermined clinical setting which will reflect a slightly different emphasis on the care of the partially sighted patient than that of the training program.

A Specific Curriculum

A specific curriculum[6] as it might appear in a college catalogue, appears in the Appendix. The curriculum itself must be constantly evaluated to determine if the training received by the technician is preparing him successfully to adapt to the different levels of utilization to which he is exposed.

At present, the demand for this type of paraprofessional is quite low. By necessity then, these training programs will be developed from existing optometric technician or ophthalmic assistant programs in which an exposure to clinical services for the partially sighted is possible. As the contributions which the technicians can make to the clinical program are realized, the demand for their services will increase.

Continuing Education Program

While a two-year training program provides technicians who have

the background to do professional low vision care, not every clinic needs or can afford to hire a full-time technician. Many clinics already depend on a competent staff member to fill a dual role. In several clinical settings today there are a number of individuals providing some of those services that the technician is properly trained to perform. They usually perform quite adequately in the dual roles they play. Nurses, social workers, mobility instructors, assistants, opticians, and educators provide services ranging from chairside assistance to ophthalmic opticians. Reviewing their contributions to their respective programs and recognizing their background, it is important to consider the possibility of providing educational programs for these people in order to give them supplementary training in optics, diagnostic tests, and low vision treatment. Obviously the answer is not in a full-fledged two-year training program but in short, intensive, goal-directed instruction.

The major low vision clinics involved in training programs must be able to provide an individualized *referral* program to train these people of different backgrounds. A short *internship* ranging from a few days to a week at a recognized training clinic could offer refresher courses depending on the needs and priorities of the applicant.

A home-study course might be worked out by the Low Vision Clinical Society, the Low Vision Diplomate Program of the Academy of Optometry, and the continuing education division of the American Academy of Ophthalmology.

Summary

In addition to decreasing the examiner's work load and allowing more patients to receive services, the technician's greatest contribution is in providing a better extended-care treatment program. The number of contact hours spent with the patient in diagnosis, training, and follow-up can be substantially increased by utilizing the low vision technician's services. This is particularly true and important in large clinic situations in which a doctor is not always available. With a technician on duty, the patient does not have to be scheduled according to the examiner's availability. Patient care can be a continuing process. Since the technician is in the examining room and participates in the doctor's determination of the prescription, the doctor's treatment program will be reflected in the technician's handling of subsequent patient visits. Through this interaction with the technician, the examiner can modify his present treatment and/or design a new program to meet the patient's needs.

When properly utilized, the technician provides a significant contribution to the low vision examination. As more clinics include the technician on their staff, the necessity for this aspect of professional service in any clinical program will be realized.

REFERENCES

1. *Vital and Health Statistics*, no. (HSM) 73-1804, ser. 14, no. 9, National Center for Health, May, 1973.
2. Loring, Philip J.: Optometric technicians and physician's assistants: new development in health care manpower: *J Am Optom Assn,* 42(5): 464-69, 1971.
3. American Optometric Association: Visual care for the 1970s: a plan for development of an optometric paraprofessional training program. St. Louis, 1971.
4. Bates, Steven S.: Paraoptometric personnel. *J Am Optom Assn,* 43(7): 774-81, 1972.
5. Cholden, Louis: *A Psychiatrist Works with Blindness.* New York, American Foundation for the Blind, 1967.
6. Optometric Technicians Program, Regional Technical Institute, University of Alabama Medical Center, 1973.

APPENDIX: CURRICULUM

Low Vision Technician Professional Curriculum

Entrance Requirements (leading to A.S. degree)

English	10 hours
Literature	5 hours
Algebra	5 hours
Physics (Survey)	5 hours
Psychology	5 hours
Speech	3 hours
Orientation to Health Occupations	3 hours
HPR	3 hours
Human Physiology/Anatomy	5 hours
Typing	3 hours

Bookkeeping 3 hours
Sociology 5 hours

These courses are taken before entering the Optometric Technician or Ophthalmic Assistant program. They are designed to introduce the student to the sciences and to prepare them for the more technical courses of the professional program.

Professional Curriculum (leading to the O.T. degree)

1st Quarter

1. Introduction and Orientation: a study of the background of optometry and the optometric technician, orientation on duties, working conditions, salaries, and job opportunities. Also included in this course is an extensive ophthalmic vocabulary orientation.
2. Anatomy and Physiology of the Eye: a study of structures and functions of the human eye, basic anatomy of the eye, and the optics of the human eye.
3. Ophthalmic Optics I: Principles of optics and how lenses and prisms correct visual problems. Techniques in laying out, cutting, edging, and verification of prescriptions. Instruction on the use of lensometer, lens clock, and ordering from the laboratory. In this course the student sees what goes into the making of an Rx, and the quality that should be expected from a local lab.
4. Preclinic practice: application of techniques for doing case history, acuity, visual fields, color vision screening, stereo screening, interpupillary distance, keratometry and tonometry.

2nd Quarter

1. Ethics and Professional Roles: The relationships in the eye care field and the roles of each member. Ethics regarding patient information. The interaction between optometry and the medical professions including referral systems and availability of social services.
2. Ophthalmic Optics II: a study in dispensing, selecting, repair and adjusting of ophthalmic frames. A continuation of Ophthalmic Optics I.

3. Clinic Patient Management: An introduction to clinical procedures in the School of Optometry Clinic and other affiliated facilities. Special emphasis is placed on applying these procedures and principles to an optometric office.
4. Clinic I: Clinical practice with senior optometry students in main clinic and affiliated clinics (low vision). Students work with senior optometry students in a doctor/technician relationship in clinical situation under supervision of clinical faculty instructor. This is the student's first exposure to the low vision patient.

3rd Quarter

1. Contact Lens Theory and Practice: Theory and optics of contact lenses, verification of contacts, teaching patients on methods of insertion and removal and hygiene as related to contacts, instrumentation and modification of contact lenses.
2. Practice Management: Effective office managing, recall systems, telephone technique, bookkeeping, peg board accounting, laboratory control, patient management.
3. Clinic II: continuation of Clinic I with emphasis on low vision patients' care. Technician will be given greater responsibilities in diagnostic and treatment aspects of the low vision examination. Identification, neutralization, and basic optics of optical aids. Introduction to low vision literature, administrative agencies dealing with blind services, and nonoptical aids.
4. Binocular Vision: an in-depth survey of the binocular visual system, orthoptics, developmental vision and clinical management of patients with binocular vision problems. Instruction on use of binocular vision testing and training equipment.

4th Quarter

Internship: advanced clinical experience in an established low vision clinical program outside of the training program. An ideal setting for the internship in this case would be a clinic with a strong ophthalmological emphasis.

INDEX

A

Aberration of lenses, 57, 59, 60, 61
Absorptive lenses
    achromatopsia, 127-128
    albinism, 128
    aphakia, 34
    brown filter, 155
    glaucoma, 155
    gray filter, 147, 153
    macular pathology, 147
    microphthalmos, 149
    Photogray, 149, 154
    retinitis pigmentosa, 155
    telescope, tinted, 192
    toxic amblyopia, 153
    Trutone, 128
    yellow filter, 155
Accommodation, 120
Achromatopsia, 127-128
Acuity, *see* Visual acuity
Acuity charts
    distance, 123
        children, 122, 123, 124, 125
    near, 123
        symbol charts, 123, 125
    reading tests, 131, 172
Acuity testing, in children, *see* Symbol test, *see also* Visual acuity
Add
    aphakia, 34, 35
    bifocal, *see* Bifocal lenses
    children, 120, 121
    related to acuity, 6
Adjustment
    to adventitial sight impairment, 5, 117, 138, 142, 165, 173, 234, 235, 236, 244, 249, 250, 257
    to congenital sight impairment, 117
Adrian, Robert J., vii, 130-136
Aging
    characteristics, 169
    Chicago Lighthouse statistics, 174, 175

funded programs, *see* Coney Island Hospital, New York
    group therapy, 165, 167, 175
    low vision examination in, 170, 171
    New York Lighthouse services,
        back-up services, 162
        community inservice, 162
        educational services, 163
        program direction, 162
    New York Lighthouse statistics,
        age groups, 159, 160
        characteristics, 161
        economic group, 161
        mobility, 161
        visual acuity, 159, 160
    prognostic factors, 173-175
    psychological factors, 170, 171, 173
    suggested reading list, 175, 176
Aids, *see* Lenses, *see also* Loan lenses, *see also* Magnifiers, Spectacles, Telescopes
    multiple, 5, 156, 173
Alabama, *see* Clinics, low vision
Albinism, 128
    astigmatism in, 128
    contact lenses in, 128
    lighting in, 128
American Optical Company, xv, 7, 10, 35, 51-59, 60, 261, 262
Amblyopia
    absorptive lenses in, 153
    prevention of, 120
    telescopes in, 153
    toxic, 153
AOlite, 10, 35, 261
Aphakia, 31-35
    aphakic refracting kit, 31-33
    cataracts, *see* Cataract, adult, *see also* Cataract, congenital
    contact lenses in, 35
    correction of, 31-35
    half-eye glasses in, 35
    high reading adds in, 35
    lighting in, 34

magnification in, 35
minimal effective diameter, 33, 34
tinted lenses for, 34
Appointments, 229, 231, 235, 237, 238, 242, 245, 257
Ary loupe, 223, 224
as carrier for telescope, 26, 27
Asarkof, John E., vii, 236-240
Aspheric, see Lenses
Astigmatism, 57
in albinism, 128

B

Barnert, Alan H., vii, 177-178, 208-211
Base-in prism, see also Prism
half-eye glass, 7, 9, 35, 156
Berens, Conrad, xi
Bifocal lenses, acceptance, 34
cataract, 34, 35
children, 120, 121, 129
congenital cataract, 120, 128, 129
hand magnifier with, 9
high adds, 10, 35, 149
indications for, 34
monocular use, 35
types, 10, 35
Binocular corrections,
add, see Half-eye glasses
telescopes, see also Telescopes
Bioptic telescopes
alignment, 21, 28, 190, 191
binocular use, 21, 190
Bioptic I, 20
binocular use, 21
characteristics, 60
driving, 20, 187
field, 20, 206
Bioptic II, 20
binocular use, 21
characteristics, 20
driving, 187
field, 20, 206
Bioptic 3X, 20, 21
characteristics, 20, 21
driving, 180, 187
field, 20, 21, 185, 200
working distance, 26
Bioptic 4X, 21
driving, 187

field, 21
Bioptic 6X, 21
field, 21
driving experience, 186, 187
driving with, 20, 28, 29, 180, 181, 186, 189, 191, 192, 194
fields in, 61, 62, 185, 200, 206
fitting of, 21, 190, 191
illustrations of, 21, 29, 61, 62, 63
ring scotoma with, 191, 205, 206
training for driving with, 194, 195
wide angle 2.2X, 20
fields of, 63, 200, 206
wide angle 3X, 21
fields of, 63
Blindness
interpretation of, 137
legal, 137, 217
variables, 137
Braille
unnecessary use of, 118
Brain damage
in children, 126, 133

C

Cataract, see also Aphakia
adult,
lens choice, 7
tinted lenses in, 34, 128
congenital, 128, 129
acuity range, 128
bifocal add, 128
braille, 118
early correction in, 118
importance of refraction, 118, 120, 128
with aphakia, 118, 120
spectacle correction, 118
surgery, 74, 75
phacoemulsification, 75
Charles, Norman C., vii, 79-86
Charts for vision testing,
see Acuity charts
Children, low vision, 117-129
achromatopsia, 127-128
accommodation in, 120
acuity testing, 119, 123
amblyopia prevention, 120
aphakia, see Cataract, congenital

Index

astigmatism, 128
bifocal, 121
brain damage in, 126, 133
case histories, 118, 119, 120, 121, 127, 128, 129
cataract, *see* Cataract, congenital
closed circuit television for, 37-41, 130-136
cycloplegia, 119, 120, 126
deafness, acuity testing in, 123
educational concepts in, 117
eye diseases, *see* disease entity
history taking, 118, 119
learning disabilities, 118, 126, 133, 134
lens types, 118, 121, 128
  bifocals, 120, 121
  contacts, 120, 128
lighting, reduced, 127, 128
low vision devices in,
  closed circuit television, 39-41
  magnifiers, hand, 121
  spectacles, 120, 121, 129
  telescopes, 121, 127
microphthalmos, 148-149
myopia, *see* Myopia
psychological testing
  closed circuit television for, 132, 133, 134
reading skills, 118
reading without glasses, 121, 127
recommendations for braille, 118
refraction in, 119, 120
retrolental fibroplasia, *see* Retrolental fibroplasia
success with aid, 129
telescopes for, 121, 127
tinted lenses, 127, 128, *see also* Absorptive lenses
visual function in, 117
Wechsler Intelligence Scale, 134
Choroiditis, 121
Clinics, low vision
Alabama, University of Alabama, School of Optometry,
  Clinic Services for the Partially Sighted, 241-252
    appendix, case history, 246-249
    appendix, report form, 251, 252
    appendix, social work evaluation, 249, 250
    appointments, 242, 245
    case history, 242
    demonstration of aids, 243
    diagnostic, 242
    examination, 242-246
    followup care, 246
    instruction, 241, 243, 244, 245, 246
    loan, 243, 244, 245
    optometric assistant, 241, 243, 244, 245, 246
    posthistory, 244
    prescription, 243
    progress history, 245
    registration fee, 241
    social worker, 244, 245
    summary report, 246, 251, 252
    technician, 241, 243, 244, 245, 246
list of low vision clinics, 216
Massachusetts, Massachusetts Eye and Ear Infirmary, Low Vision Center, 267-272
  Boston Aid to the Blind, 268
  Carroll Rehabilitation Center, 268
  examination, 268
  Nightscope, 271
  ophthalmologist, 268, 269
  optometrist, 268, 269, 271
  patient interview, 270, 271
  program coordination, 271
  referral, 272
  referral source, 270
  resident training, 267-272
  staff, 268
  technician training, 268, 269
  training program, 268
University Hospital, Vision Rehabilitation Clinic, 228-240
  appointments, 229, 231, 235, 237, 238
  community program, 228
  counseling, 230, 234, 235
  development, 233
  film, 240
  followup, 231, 235, 238
  funding, 229

goals, 228
group counseling, 236
loan system, 229, 230, 237, 238
ophthalmologist, 228-232
optometrist, 228, 236-240
records, 239
referral sources, 231
social worker, 231, 234-236
staff, 229, 239
statistics, 228
student teaching, 232, 233, 235, 237
New York, Lighthouse Low Vision Service, 253-263
appointments, 257
assistant, low vision, 254, 255, 256
case histories, 259, 260
examination, 255
instruction, 256, 257
instruction room, 256
failure, 257, 258
followup, 257
loan system, 254, 258-263
cost, 263
equipment, 260, 261
lens inventory, 261, 262
lens maintenance, 262
lens storage, 262
lenses most loaned, 262
rationale for, 258, 259, 263
statistics 258, 259, 262
New York, Rochester Association for the Blind, Low Vision Clinic, 220-227
aids used, 223, 224, 227
case histories, 225, 226
community programs, 222, 223
counseling, 227
development of the clinic, 220-222
funding, 222
pathology examined, 225
problems, administrative, 223-225, 226
referral sources, 221, 225, 226
staff, 221
statistics, aids prescribed, 223, 224
success, 223

number of clinics, 216
organizational problems, 215-216
statistics, legally blind, 217
partially sighted, 217
Closed circuit television, 37-41, 130-136
advantages, 37, 38
Bender test on, 132, 134
case histories, 39-41, 135
components, 38
development, 38
intelligence tests, 134
lighting, 38
magnification, 37
music, 40, 41, 135
psychological tests, 132, 134
reading speed, 135
reading tests, 132, 133
rehabilitation aid, 38
retinitis pigmentosa, 135
uveitis, 154
Wechsler intelligence scale for children, 134
Color vision, 127
Community Services, see also Clinics, Low vision
Alabama
University of Alabama, Clinical Services for the Partially Sighted, viii, 241-252
California
Southern California College of Optometry, Low Vision Service, viii
Illinois
Chicago Lighthouse, Low Vision Clinic, 169-176, ix
Massachusetts
Massachusetts Eye and Ear Infirmary, Low Vision Center, viii, 267-272
University Hospital, Vision Rehabilitation Clinic, viii, 228-240
Michigan
Sinai Hospital, Low Vision Service, viii, 37-41
New York
Coney Island Hospital, see Coney Island Hospital

Index

Industrial Home for the Blind, Low Vision Service, vii
Nassau County Medical Center, Low Vision Resident Program, ix
New York Association for the Blind, Lighthouse Low Vision Service, vii, viii
   agency services, 137-140, 141-145, 159-163
   low vision services, 130-136
   Rochester Association for the Blind, Low Vision Clinic, 220-227, vii
Pennsylvania, Wills Eye Hospital Low Vision Aid Service, ix
Coney Island Hospital, New York
   funded programs for elderly blind, 166
   continuing education, 167
   counseling services, 165, 167
   geriatric demonstration program, 164
   group resocialization, 165
   medical services, 165
   nutritional program, 165
   therapeutic recreation, 165
   transportation, 165
   vision screening, 166
   volunteer training, 166
Contact lens, see Aphakia, see also Children, lens types, see also, Lenses, contact, see also Telescope
Convex lenses
   characteristics, 51, 52
   effective power, 51, 55
   equiconvex lenses, 56, 57
   equivalent power, 54
   optical design, 51-59
   plano convex, 56, 58
Corneal disease, case history, 154
Crossed cylinders, 171

D

Designs for Vision, 20, 21, 60, 63
   Bioptic telescope, see Bioptic telescopes
   telemicroscope, 27
Diabetic equipment, see Non-optical

Diabetes mellitus, see also, Laser, macula
   aids for diabetics, 47
   rehabilitation, 137
Diabetic retinopathy
   absorptive lenses in, 155
   case history, 155
   lens choice, 7
   macula, 82, 83
   neck magnifier for, 155
   telescopic correction for, 155
   treatment, laser, 83, 89, 90
Diagnosis, confirmation of, 98, 102, 129
Dioptric power
   of convex spheres, 51-59
   related to focal distance, 52, 54
   of stand magnifiers, 15
   true dioptric power, 54-58
Directory of Services
   Directory of Agencies Serving the Visually Handicapped in the U.S., American Foundation for the Blind, 173
Diseases of the eye, see under individual disease entity
Distance lenses, see Lenses, distance
Distance vision, see Visual acuity
Driving
   acuity standards, 179, 180, 183, 184, 187, 199, 200, 204
   Bioptic in, 180, 181, 185, 186, 187, 189, 204
   compact car for low vision drivers, 192
   criteria for licensure
      American Medical Association, 183, 184
      Kelleher and Korb, 189, 193, 205
      low vision candidates, 180, 187
      Massachusetts, 188
      New York, 199, 201
      North Carolina, 179
      Pennsylvania, 204
   evaluation, professional
      Department of Motor Vehicles, 195, 196, 198, 201, 203
   experience, 186, 187
   fatalities, 181, 196, 197, 204
   field, peripheral, 200

glare, 192
illumination factors, 192, 194
mirror
  rear view, 206
  side view, 180, 191, 201
necessity, 179, 189, 208
parallax, telescopic, 101
problems, 191, 192, 205, 206, 209
recommendations, 209
  against driving, 205
  safety, 193
research, 180, 210
safety record
  drivers' statements, 187
  Indiana State Police, 184
  Massachusetts, 181, 185, 197
scotoma, ring, 191, 202, 203, 205, 206
standards for driving, 28, 178
standard transmission, 192
success, 185
telescopes in, 20, 28, 29
  fields, 185
  fitting, 190, 191
test, telescope in, 206
training procedures, 180, 181, 193, 194, 195
visual field standards, 180, 184, 187, 189
vibration, affecting acuity, 191 206, 207
Dyslexia, *see* Learning disabilities

E

Educational evaluation, 118
Electroretinography, 72
Equipment
  aphakic refracting kit, 31-33
  charts for vision testing, 122, 125
  clinic supplies, 256, 260, 261
  closed circuit television, 38
  Halberg clip, 35, 172
  Lighthouse magnifier kit, 34
  loan lenses, 260, 261, 262
  non-optical devices, 42-48, 254
  optokinetic drum, 123, 124, *see also* Nonoptical visual aids
  trial sets, 10

F

Failure
  definition, 259
  depression, 139
  disadvantages of magnification, 6, 10, 51
  factors in, 137, 142
  limitations of lenses, 42, 48, 51
  medical, 139
  poor vision, 139
  reducing failure, 235, 238, 239, 244, 245, 246, 263
  rejection of lenses, 140, 51
  statistical analysis, 258
Faye, Eleanor E., vii, xi, 5-16, 253-263
Feinbloom, Richard E., vii, 60-68
Field defects
  central, 97
  hemianopia, 98, 99, 101, 103, 104, 108
  neurological, 98
  in vocational planning, 99
  peripheral, 97, 103, 104, 105
  prism in, 99, 103-113
Fields, telescopic, *see* Bioptic telescopes, *see also* Keeler, *see also* Selsi, *see also* Wide angle telescope
Field of vision, *see* Field defects, *see also* Scotomas, *see also* Visual fields
Films, 240, 275
Fine, Leslie, vii, 164-168
Focal distance, *see* Lenses, working distance
  convex spheres, 51-59
Focal point, definition, 64
Followup, 144, 231, 235, 238, 239, 246, 257, 259, 279
Fonda, Gerald, xi, 206
Forms, case history, 246
  followup, 239
  report forms, 251, 252
  social work evaluation, 249
Formulas,
  diopters of reading add, 6
  dioptric power, 52
  focal distance of convex lenses, 54, 57
  guide to strength of aid, 226, 227
  magnification, 55

Index

Frames
  alignment, importance of, 128
  aphakia, 32, 33, 34
  Bioptic alignment, 21, 28, 190
  flip-up, 199, 200
Fresnel prisms, 7, 106, 113
  advantages, 106
  adds for aphakia, 35
  application of, 104, 106, 108
  base, 104, 105, 108
  characteristics, 104, 107
  cost, 106
  field movement, 104
  field widening effect, 105
  indications, 99, 104, 105, 109
  limitations, 109
  optical characteristics, 106, 107
  prism power, 104, 105, 108, 109
  rejection, 106
  retinitis pigmentosa, 104, 105, 110, 111
  removal, 108
  reuse, 108
  use, 99, 106
Friedman, Dagmar B., vii, 234-236

G

Galilean telescope, definition of, 17
  see also, Telescopes
  characteristics, 18
  working distance, 26
Glaucoma
  case history, 40
  field, 97
  lens choice, 14
Gordon, Arlene R., vii, 159-163
Gruber, Ellis, vii, 220-227

H

Halberg clip, 35, 172
Half-eye glasses, 7-9, 156
  in aphakia, 35
  nasal field loss, 155, 156
Hand magnifiers, see Magnifiers, hand-held
Hellinger, George O., vii, 146-156, 199-203
Hemianopia, see Visual fields, see also Scotomas

History taking
  in adults, 170, 171, 234, 242, 244, 245, 253, 270, 271
  in children, 118, 119
  timing of history, 253
Hoeft, Wayne W., viii, 103-113
Hood, Clare M., viii, 42-48, 253-263
Hyperactivity, 147

I

Illiterates, vision test for, 122, 123, 125
Illuminated magnifiers, 15
Illumination, see Lighting, see also, Driving
Illustrations
  fields, hemianopia, 101, 104
    peripheral loss, 108
  fields of telescopes, 65, 66, 67, 202, 203
  Fresnel prism, 106, 107, 113
  half-eye glasses, 7
  hemianopic mirror, 105, 112
  inferior hemianopia, 100
  lens characteristics, 52, 53, 56, 57, 58
  macular area, 98
  magnifiers, hand, 8, 10, 11, 12, stand, 13, 14, 15
  near vision test card, 125
  neck magnifier, 16, 156
  non-optical, 43
  optokinetic drum, 124
  peripheral field loss, 99
  prism effect, 107
  prism in retinitis pigmentosa, 110, 111
  records, 239, 251, 252
  retina, normal, 81
  retina, diabetic, 83
  retina, treated, 83
  retrolental fibroplasia, 148
    using intermediate telescope, 151
    reading with 8X spectacle, 149
    using 1.7X telescope, 150
    using 6X monocular, 152
  telescopes
    Bioptic, 21, 29, 61, 62, 63
    flip-up frame, 200

Keeler, 23, 27
Selsi, 22, 24
telemicroscope, 27, 153
visual acuity symbols, 122
Intermediate vision, correction of, 29, 61, 151, 154, 190
see also Keeler

J

"Jack-in-the-box" hazard, 205-206, *see also,* Scotoma, ring
Jaeger test type, 35, 225, 226
Jose, Randall T., viii, 215-219, 241-252, 276-284

K

Keeler
clip-on occluder, 9
crescent lenses for reading, 9
ring telescope, 23
telemicroscope, 25-27
Keeney, Arthur H., viii, 204-207
Kelleher, Dennis K., viii, 189-198
Keratoplasty, 72-73
Kestenbaum, Alfred, xi
formula, 6
Kraut, Joel A., viii, 267-272
Kuhns, Thomas R., viii, 97-102

L

Large print, 9, 48, 120
point size, 118, 120, 125, 128, 129, *see also* Non-optical
Learning disabilities 118, 126, 133, 134
Laser
Argon, 80, 87-93
in central serous retinopathy, 90, 91
contraindications to treatment, 90, 92
diseases, treatable, 88, 90
effect, 80, 91, 92
evaluation of patient, 88
histoplasmosis, treatment, 93
macula
anatomical principles, 81, 82
diffuse macular abnormalities, 82

diabetes, 82
exudative diseases, 82, 92
local vascular abnormalities of, 84
non-exudative disease, 91
prognosis, 85, 92
secondary disorders, 82
treatment, 84, 92
pigment epithelium detachments, 91
properties of, 87
response to magnification after treatment, 92
retinal proliferative disease, 89, 90
therapeutic considerations, 79, 80, 87, 89, 90, 91, 92
vascular proliferative disease, 90
venous occlusive disease, 88, 89
Legal blindness, *see* Blindness
Lenses
aberrations in, 57, 59, 60, 61
absorptive, *see* Absorptive lenses
afocal, *see* Telescopes
aphakic corrections, 31-36
aspheric, 31, 33, 34, 35, 59, 60
astigmatism, 57
bifocal, *see* Bifocal
carrier lens, *see* Telescopes
characteristics, 52, 53, 56, 57, 58
convex, *see* Convex lenses
cylinder, *see* Astigmatism
definition, 51
design, 51-59
dioptric power, 52
distance lenses
aphakic, 31-35
aspheric, 31, 33, 34, 35, 60
bifocal, indications for, 34, 35
concave, *see* Myopia
contact lenses
aphakic corrections, 35
in congenital cataracts with aphakia, 120 128
telescope, 24, 25
doublet, 60, 61
effective power, 51, 55
equivalent focal length, 54
equivalent power, 52-54, 55
focal distance, *see* Lenses, working distance
Fresnel, 7, *see also* Fresnel

full vision glasses, 9
lensometer power, 55-57
loan lenses, *see* Loan lenses
low vision lenses, *see* Magnifiers,
   see also Spectacles, *see also*
   Telescopes
magnification, *see* Magnification
magnifiers, *see* Magnifiers
magnifying power, 54, 55
near vision lenses
   AOlite, 10
   aspheric, 59
   bifocal, *see* Bifocal lenses
   calculating add, 6
   definition of low vision lenses, 5
   focal distance, convex spheres,
     52-54
   half-eye glasses, 7-9, 35
   hand magnifiers, *see* Magnifiers,
     hand-held
   optical aids, *see* Optical aids
   prism, 7, *see also* Prism
   spectacles, *see* Spectacles
   stand magnifiers, *see* Magnifiers,
     stand magnifiers
plastic, properties of, 62, 63
prism, *see* Fresnel, *see also* Prism
reading field of lenses, 9, 51
spectacle, *see* Spectacles
successful aids, 175
telescopes, *see* Telescopes
trial lenses, 6, 9
true dioptric power, 54-58
working distance, 6, 9, 10, 13, 26,
   27, 54, 56, 57, 58, 59, 64, 172
Lighthouse Low Vision Service, *see*
   New York Lighthouse Low
   Vision Service
magnifier kit, 34
optical aids catalogue, 16
optical aids service, 263
rehabilitation, 139, 140, 144, 163,
   see also Aging
test cards, 123
   illustrations of vision cards, 124,
     125
service statistics, 159, 160, 161
Lighting, 15, 38, 42, 127, 128, 155,
   171, 172
   closed circuit television source, 38

effects of glare, 46
illuminated stand, 15
illumination
   appropriate, 34, 171
   for drivers with low vision,
     192, 194
   effects of bright light, 155
   effects of reduced light, 127, 128
   as non-optical aid, 42, 44
Loan lenses, 229, 230, 237, 238, 243,
   244, 245, 254, 258-263
Low vision, *see* Clinics, low vision
   adjustment to, 138, 236
   attitudes towards, 140
   counseling, 139, 140, 230, 234, 235
   defined, 5, 217
   as disability, driving, 179
   evaluation, 139
   examination, 6, 7, 139, 141,
     242-246, 255
   failure, 137, 142, 174, 257
   followup, 144, 231, 235, 237, 238,
     246
   forms, *see* Forms
   inservice seminar, 217, 218
   instruction, 244, 245, 246, 256, 257
   loan system, 229, 230, 237, 238,
     243, 244, 245, 254, 258-265
   manpower shortage in eye care, 215
   orientation and mobility in, 173
   psychological evaluation, 173
   range of acuity, 137
   rehabilitation in, 138, 139, 140,
     142, 143, 144
   staff interaction, 140, 141, 144,
     229, 230, 233, 239, 271
Low vision assistant, *see* Low vision
   technician,
   New York Lighthouse, 254, 255;
     256
   training program, 280, 281
Low vision clinic, *see* Clinics, low
   vision
Low vision Lenses, *see* Lenses, *see*
   also Magnifiers, *see also* Spectacles,
   see also Telescopes
Low vision technicians, training,
   276-284, 268, 269
   continuing education, 280-281
   internship, 281

suggested course, 281
types of applicants, 281
curriculum, 280, 282-284
   1st quarter, 283
   2nd quarter, 283-284
   3rd quarter, 284
   4th quarter, 284
definition, 277, 281-282
entrance requirements, 282
training program, 277-280
   diagnostic procedure, 278
   internship, 280, 284
   introduction to examination, 278
   orientation to low vision, 278
   training and followup, 279

M

Macular pathology, *see also* Laser
   acuity, 97, 98
   case history, 39, 146
   central scotoma, 97
   central serous choroidopathy, 90, 91
   diabetic, 82, 83
   edema, 82, 84, 89, 90
   lens choice, 7
   normal, 81
   prognosis, 85
   proliferative disease, 85, 89, 90
   senile maculopathy, 84, 91, 92
   treatment of, 85, 88, 89, 90
   zones, 98
Magnification
   in aphakia, 35
   closed circuit television, 37
   definition in low vision, 82, 84
   formulas for, 54, 55
   telescopic, 18, 19, 22, 23, 25
Magnifiers
   advantages, 10, 12
   available aids, 12, 14, 15
   chest magnifier, *see* Magnifiers, stand magnifiers
   field of magnifiers, 9, 10
   focal distance, 6, 9, 10, 13
   formula for prescription, *see* Formula
   hand-held magnifiers
      as alternative to spectacles, 8, 10-13

      in aphakia, 34
      characteristics, 10, 15
      in children, 121
      with constricted fields, 14
      focal length, 10
      in glaucoma, 14
      with half-eye glass, 9
      for increased reading distance, 13
      for intermediate area, 13
      optical properties, 10, 15
      strengths of, 11-15
      as training device, 7, 13
      types of, 7-15
      uses of, 13
   stand magnifiers, 13, 14-16
      characteristics, 14, 15
      chest magnifier, 15, 16, 156
      fixed focus, 15
      illuminated, 15
      light gathering properties, 15
Massachusetts, Boston *see* Clinics, low vision
   Massachusetts Eye and Ear Infirmary, Low Vision Center
   University Hospital, Vision Rehabilitation Clinic
McAdams, LoRetta, viii, 241-252
McDonald, Kay, viii, 141-145
Medow, Norman B., viii, 71- 78
Mintz, Morris, viii, 37-41
Microphthalmos, 148-149
Mirrors,
   cosmetic effect in hemianopia, 105, 106
   hemianopia, 99, 103, 104, 105, 112
   rear view, 206
   side view, 180, 191, 201
   use of in driving, 191, 193, 196
Monocular, *see also* Telescopes
   binoculars used as monocular, 25
   occlusion, 9, 260
   reading, 35
   in retrolental fibroplasia, 126
Moore, Charles, viii, 31-36
Myopia
   case histories, 119, 120, 121, 127
   reading without correction, 8, 127
   refraction in, 127

Index

N

Near vision, *see* Visual acuity, near
Near vision lenses, *see* Lenses, near vision
Near vision testing
 test charts, 123, 125
 see also Visual acuity, near
Neurological examination
 importance of, 102
 visual fields in, 97-102
Newman, Julian D., viii, 17-30, 179-182
New York Association for the Blind, xi-xv, *see also* New York Lighthouse Low Vision Service
New York Lighthouse Low Vision Service, *see* Clinics, low vision
New York, Rochester Low Vision Clinic, *see* Clinics, low vision
Night blindness, 271
 poor night vision, 204
Night driving, 201, 205
Nightscope, 271
Non-optical visual aids, 42-48
 cards, 46
 definition of, 42
 diabetic equipment, 47
 illustration, 43
 large print, 48
 lighting, 42, 44
 reading material, 48
 reading stands, 46, 47
 sewing aids, 45, 46
 telephone dial, 45
 writing material, 44, 45
Nystagmus
 in achromatopsia, 102, 128
 in albinism, 102, 128
 in children, 126
 in congenital cataract, 129
 differential diagnosis, 102
 head position, minimizing, 126
 in retrolental fibroplasia, 127
 significance of, 102

O

Occlusion of lens, 9, 260
Occupational needs, *see* Vocational needs
Optical aids, *see* Magnifiers, *see also* Spectacles, *see also* Telescopes, *see also* Optical Aids Service
Optical Aids Service, xii, 263
 Lighthouse Optical Aids Catalogue, 16
Optic atrophy
 accurate diagnosis, 102
 case histories, 39, 40, 41
 causes of, 102
 field of vision, 98
Optokinetic drum, 123
 illustration, 124

P

Partial sight, *see* Low vision
Photophobia
 in achromatopisia, 127, 128
 in albinism, 128, 192
Press-on prism, *see* Fresnel prism
Prism, *see* Base-in prism, *see also* Lenses, prism base-in
 see also Fresnel prism
Prosthokeratoplasty, 73, 74
Psychological
 evaluation in aged, 173
 factors, in aged, 170, 171, 173
 tests on closed circuit television, 132, 134

R

Reading
 cap for telescope, 27, 29, 68
 in closed circuit television, *see* closed circuit television
 difficulty, 97, 98, 99
 efficiency, 39-41
 field, 97
 music, 41, 135
 problems in children, 118
 reading distance, *see* Lenses, focal length, working distance
 reading references on aged, 175-176
 speed, 39, 135
 tests on CCTV, 132, 133
Reading field, *see* Spectacles
Refraction
 aphakic, 31-35

children, 119, 120
cross cylinder, 171
cycloplegic, 119, 120, 126
in elderly patients, 171-173
high errors of, 172
importance of, 172
phoropter, 126
Rehabilitation
adaptation, 142
definition, 141
case history, 142
closed circuit television in, 38, 39
community participation, 162, 165, 166, 167
community services, see Clinics, low vision, see also Community services
follow-up, 144, 231, 235, 238, 239, 246, 257, 259, 279
geriatric population, see Aging, see also Coney Island Hospital, New York
low vision prescription, 140, 144
procedures, 139, 140
subgroups of clients
established adults, 138, 164, 165
losing current job, 139
most impaired, 139
needing single service only, 138
retaining present job, 138, 143
staff interaction, 140, 141, 144, 165, 167, 217, 218
trends, 137
use of residual vision in, 143
Resident training, 267-272, 273-275
basic science course, 274
films, 275
literature, 275
Residual vision, see Low vision
Retinitis pigmentosa
absorptive lenses in, 155
case history, 40, 135
closed circuit television as aid, 135
field defect in, 97, 103, 104, 105, 108
Nightscope, 271
night vision, 271
prisms as aid, 104, 105, 110, 111
Retinopathies, vascular, 79-86, 87-93
contraindications to treatment, 90, 92

description of,
exudative, 89, 92
hemorrhagic, 92
proliferative, 90
prognosis, 89, 90, 91, 92
treatment, 89, 92
Retrolental fibroplasia
case history, 39, 127, 147, 148
description of behavior, 147
refraction, 126, 127
telescopic devices, 147, 149, 150, 151, 152
Rosenbloom, Alfred A., ix, 169-176

S

Scotomas, see Field defects
as factor in reading difficulties, 97, 99
in glaucoma, 97
hemianopia, 98, 99, 103, 104, 108
in macular pathology, 97
in optic atrophy, 98
prisms in, see Fresnel prisms, see also Hemianopia, see also Retinitis pigmentosa
in retinitis pigmentosa, 97, 103, 104, 105
ring, 191, 205, 206, see also "Jack-in-the-box" hazard
Seidenberg, Boyd H., ix, 117-129
Selsi, 12, 14, 21, 22, 23, 24, 25, 35, 262, 263
telescope strengths
2.5X, 22
2.8X, 22
6X-8X, 21, 23, 35
10X, 24
Zoom, 24, 25
Sprague, Wesley D., xii
Spectacles
advantages, 10
bifocals, see Lenses, bifocal
binocular corrections, see Lenses binocular
cataracts, correction of, see Lenses, see also Aphakia
characteristics, 9, 51
children, 117-129
distance correction, see Lenses, distance
fields, reading, 9, 10, 51

focal distance, 6, 9
formula for add, *see* Formula
full vision, 9
indications, 9
half-eye, 7, 9
limitation, 10
loan lenses, *see* Loan lenses
magnification principle, 54, 55
monocular occlusion, 9
optical characteristics, 51-59
premounted, 9
prism, *see* Prism, *see also*
  Fresnel prism
reading field in, 9, 10, 51
for refractive error, 10, 31-35
rejection, 6
tinted, *see* Absorptive lenses
Stand magnifiers, *see* Magnifiers,
  stand magnifiers
Statistical analysis, *see also* Aging
  estimate of low vision population,
    217
  population of low vision drivers,
    197
  loan lenses, 258, 259, 262
  success and failure, 216, 258
  visual acuity requirements by
    states, 183
Stern, Elisabeth, ix, 137-140
Sterns, Gwen Kunken, ix, 273-275
Subnormal vision, *see* Low Vision
Success
  case histories, 142, 143
  factors, 137
  importance of training, 140
Sunglasses, *see* Absorptive lenses
Symbol test, Lighthouse symbol test,
  122, 123, 125
  testing children's acuity, 122, 123,
    125

T

Tables
  children
    incidence of pathology,
      1953-1968, 127
    incidence of pathology,
      1969-1972, 126
  loan lenses, 262
  ocular pathology, 225

population of low vision drivers,
  197
relationship of lens power, 55
type of aids prescribed, 224
visual acuity requirements by states,
  183
Tallman, Carter, B., ix, 183-188,
  228-233
Telemicroscopes, 25-28, 153, 154
  Designs for Vision, 27
  Keeler, 25-27
Telescopes
  afocal, 18
  binoculars, 25, 29
  binocular use, 21, 190, 191, 206
  Bioptic, 20, 21, 28, 30, 35, 187,
    191, 192, 194, 195, 204, 206
    see also Bioptic telescope
  carrier lens, 20, 27, 191, 199, 205,
    206, 209
  characteristics, 18
  children, *see* Children, telescopes
  considerations in prescribing, 28, 29
  contact lens, 24, 25
  distance refraction using, 19, 172
  driving, 20, 28, 29, 180, 181,
    186, 189-193, 200, 201, 205-207
  driving experience, 186, 187,
    189-193, 197
  field, 65, 66, 67, 202, 203, *see also*
    Bioptic telescope
  field restriction, 200, 202, 203, 206
  flip-up frames, 27, 200
  focal distance, 26
  Galilean, definition of, 17, *see also*
    Galilean telescope
  hand held, 22-24
  head borne, 20-22
  indications, 20-23, 25, 26, 28, 29
  intermediate correction, 29, 61, 151,
    153, 154, 190
  Keeler, *see* Keeler
  light transmission, 18, 25, 64
  limitations, 20
  mobility, 140
  monocular, 21-22, 23, 24, 25, 35
  occupational needs, 29
  parallax, 191
  prescription related to visual
    acuity, 28
  reading cap, 27, 29, 68

recreational needs, 29, 140
refraction with, 19, 172
reverse, 104, 105
ring, 23
scotoma, ring, 191, 205
Selsi, *see* Selsi
spotting device, 210
telemicroscope, 25-28, 153, 154
tint in, 192
unusual types, 28
wide angle, 20, 21, 180, 200, 202, 206, 261, 262
Tinted lenses, *see* Absorptive lenses
Training programs *see also* Resident training
 optometry students, 237, 241, 271
 resident, ophthalmology, 233, 267-272, 273-275
 technician, low vision, 268-269, 276-284, *see also* Low vision assistant
 social work student teaching, 232, 233, 235, 237
Trial lenses, *see* Lenses trial
Trial sets, 10, 34
True dioptric power, *see* Lenses

U

Ultrasonography, 72
Uveitis
 absorptive lenses in, 154
 aphakic correction in, 154
 closed circuit television for, 154

V

Visual acuity
 case histories, 39-41
 diffuse loss, 99
 distance vision
  aphakic correction, 31-35
  laser treatment related to, 90
  related to visual aids, 7, 9, 12, 22, 23, 28, 39-41
  test charts
   optokinetic drum, 123, 124
   Lighthouse symbol cards, 122, 123
  test distance, 171
  testing, accurate, 100, 119, 123
  used to calculate the add, 6
 glare, 46, 192

lighting, 15, 38, 42, 127, 128, 155, 171, 172
macular disease, 91, 97, 98
myopia cases, 119, 120, 121, 127
near vision, 123
 measurement, 123, 172
 related to visual aids, 92
 test charts, Lighthouse, 123, 125
 used to calculate the add, 6
 reciprocal of, 6
nystagmus, 126
range in low vision, 137
refraction in elderly, 171-173
standards for driving, 28, *see also* Driving
telescope for testing, 19, 172
Visual fields
 central loss, 97
 description of, *see* Field defects
 hemianopia, 98, 99, 101, 103, 104, 108
 mobility in, 103
 peripheral, 108, 201
 peripheral loss, 97, 99, 103, 104, 105
  lens choice in, 14, 103-113
 reading difficulty in, 97, 98, 99
 scotomas, *see* Scotomas
 telescopic, restricted, 210
Vitrectomy, 75, 76
Vocational use of,
 hand magnifiers, 143
 spectacles, 143
 telescopes, 29, 143

W

Weiss, Sidney, viii, 204-207
Welsh, Robert, 31
Whitney, Donald B., ix, 51-59
Wide angle telescope, 20, 21, 180, 200, 202, 206, 261, 262
 see also Bioptic, wide angle
Working distance, *see* Lenses

Y

Yannuzzi, Lawrence, ix, 87-93

Z

Zoom lens
 closed circuit television, 38
 monocular, 25